Praise for *Spotting Danger*

"In my twenty years on the job, I have se⟨
The world is full of victims and surviv⟨
survivor."

—Burk Stearns, MBA, BS Crim⟨
Lieutenant, Field Watch Commander,
California Court Recognized Gang Expert

"In the modern world, danger abounds and none of us are immune to the threat of it, but what does it look like and how do we recognize and avoid it? Gary Quesenberry has *forgotten* more about how to spot danger than most us will ever know. Thankfully, he remembered the most important stuff and has put it in this book! *Spotting Danger Before It Spots You* is a must-read for anyone who doesn't have the Secret Service doing their danger-spotting for them. Gary delivers no-nonsense advice on a serious and relevant topic with an engaging blend of humor, common sense, and the wisdom that comes from three decades of having lived in a world where spotting danger was a necessity."

—LCDR Jonathan Cleck, Navy Seal,
Cohost of the *Kill Cliff* podcast

"Practicing situational awareness is one of the most important things a person can do to keep themselves and others safe. I think it is the most important thing I teach in my Safety, Self-Defense, and Survive a Shooting programs. And while many books mention awareness, Gary Quesenberry actually shows you in his book how to be more aware and what to be aware of. He provides key concepts, real-world examples, and practical exercises to help you develop the attitude and situational awareness necessary to avoid most violence, and he offers solid advice for those times you can't. The three phases—Understanding the Threat, Building Your Situational Awareness, and Developing Personal Defenses—are the keys to staying safe and not becoming a victim. Practicing situational awareness will not only allow you to see potential danger early enough to do something about it, it just may mean the difference between life and death. Yes, situational awareness is that important, and this book is that important. Read it, practice situational awareness when you are out and about, and enjoy life safely."

—Alain Burrese, JD, author, fifth dan hapkido,
former army sniper

"Gary Quesenberry's book is an all-encompassing guide and essential resource for understanding how to stay safe in today's world. Gary shares proven personal safety tactics, techniques, and procedures that are taught at the highest levels of government, law enforcement, and the military.

"His proactive approach to identifying potential trouble is spot on. But he doesn't stop there. He touches upon simple and effective defense techniques specially created to be quick and effective. His real-life stories and examples of criminal activity give the lay person a road map for how to avoid being targeted in the first place.

"This is mandatory reading for those of you who wish to make yourself and your loved ones a 'hard target.'"

—Steven M. Kinsey, police firearms and tactics instructor,
US Department of Homeland Security

"There is an old saying in sports, 'The best defense is a good offense.' This is also supremely true when it comes to personal defense. So many peoples' plans and preparations for personal defense begin and end with the concealed carry of a firearm, gun fighting tactics, or martial arts. This ideal is perpetuated by the booming 'tactical industry' with its peddling of 'everyday-carry' gadgets and social media videos romanticizing the CCW Instagram quick-draw.

"This is a book that had to be written. People need to understand that making it back home safe and sound shouldn't rely on your fighting or shooting ability. The secret of self-defense is recognizing and avoiding dangerous situations altogether–which is what makes this book so brilliant."

—Jamie Franks, US Navy chief petty officer
(twenty-two year veteran), competitive shooter on
The History Channel's *Top Shot All-Stars*

"When I was sixteen, I was mugged in an isolated train station in Madrid, Spain. For years I felt ashamed that I didn't fight hard enough to save my deceased grandfather's gold necklace and cross from theft. Since then, my years of training and experience in special operations, counter-terrorism, and federal law enforcement taught me that the loss of the fight was not the true failure. It was the culmination of my mistakes which made me unaware of the imminent attack and made the two attackers view me as an easy target.

"My attire made me stand out like a foreigner, and I was sitting in an unpopulated and dark area of the station that offered few avenues of escape. I was not aware of my surroundings, and I didn't give credence to my intuition. Every mistake leading to the mugging was my choice; I wasn't a victim of a random attack. In reading Gary's book, I am reminded of these errors, but I am also reminded of the strategies I could have used to avoid them.

"I can't go back in time to that evening and apply all the principles I learned from years of law enforcement experience. But if I had read this book as a sixteen-year-old and applied its techniques, I am certain that those two muggers and I would never have had an exchange. They wouldn't have seen me as an easy target, but even if they had, I would have been able to see the attack coming.

"This book is for everyone. The inexperienced will learn how to avoid being a target, spot an attack before it happens, and form a plan of action in response, while those who are experienced in these matters will come to see areas in their lives where they have become too complacent about over the years."

—Carlos Poysky, law enforcement physical techniques instructor, Department of Homeland Security, former airborne ranger (1st Ranger Battalion, 75th Ranger Regiment 1995–1998), former air marshal and air marshal instructor

"I have known Gary Quesenberry for over fifteen years. As an adjunct instructor who worked for me and as a credentialed federal air marshal, Gary was always a top-notch instructor and operator, a complete professional who stood out among his peers. Anything Gary puts his name on is first rate, and that includes this book, which he has written at a time when real-world situational awareness is a critical skill to have. Situational awareness is the critical skill for an undercover air marshal, and his background has no doubt vastly enhanced his ability to teach his readers about the subject. In our tactics instruction, we always preached that spotting a threat versus reacting to one was the key to winning a fight at thirty-five thousand feet in a tubular aircraft with no backup, cover, or place to hide. This book is a must-read for anyone who wants to learn the skills involved in observing their environment and using what they observe to make them safer. Written in a no-fluff style, it is broken down into learnable chunks (phases) that will make every single person who opens the cover better prepared."

—Michael R. Seeklander, owner of The American Warrior Society and Shooting-Performance Training Systems, author of *Your Competition Handgun Training Program, Your Defensive Handgun Training Program, Your Defensive Rifle Training Program,* and *The Art of Instruction*

"*Spotting Danger Before It Spots You* is a book everyone who leaves the safety of their home on a daily basis should read. His book made me realize how the way I had been going about my everyday activities was making me a potential target. I learned a lot about how to harden my defenses with the exercises Gary provides."

—Gabby Franco, competitive shooter, author of *Trouble Shooting: Mastering Your Pistol Marksmanship*

"*Spotting Danger Before It Spots You* is filled with crucial information that should be passed down to those you love. Regardless of how much our world changes, humankind continues to victimize itself. This information should be incorporated into your lifestyle in order to protect yourself and others from harm. The author does a superb job of drawing principles and techniques from his life experience and communicating them to the reader in a no-nonsense writing style."

—Rod Smith, law enforcement officer,
owner of SpecGear—Tactical Concealed Carry

"Over my twenty-five-plus years in law enforcement, no subject has been more important than situational awareness. For those who serve inside the walls of America's toughest prisons, the ability to stay in tune with their surroundings is all important. This book identified traits associated with situational awareness that have become second nature for me, but I had to learn those traits on my own in the course of my career, and I wish I had had a book like this to make learning those essential skills easier. Gary's book provides an essential foundation for situational awareness, and I plan on making it required reading for officers and staff."

—Darrin McWhorter, captain in the Federal Bureau of
Prisons, Special Operations Response Team Commander,
and National Tactical Trainer

"Crime can happen to anyone, anywhere, and at any time. *Spotting Danger Before It Spots You* contains solid advice that's been, literally, proven the world over.

Gary shares his wealth of knowledge and provides real-world case studies involving personal safety and security that are applicable to the seasoned professional as well as to the average citizen. He covers the concepts involved in being aware of your surroundings and stopping a problem before it starts. Full of practical and easy-to-follow recommendations that will help keep you safe, this material Gary presents in this book will bridge any gaps in your personal planning, awareness, and understanding as either a safety professional or ordinary citizen."

—Jennifer N. Mitchell, US Department of Homeland Security,
former police officer, Lansing, Michigan

"*Spotting Danger Before It Spots You* is a must-read. Gary has written *the* manual for the average citizen on situational awareness. The skills he teaches in this book are the same skills I have used in the US Air Force, the Secret Service, and Federal Air Marshal Service. You can practice defensive measures, fighting skills, concealed carry, and verbal judo, but without knowing how to evaluate your everyday life, you are leaving a gaping hole in your defense plan."

—Gary J. Byrne, federal air marshal (Ret.), former
Air Force security policeman, secret service
(police officer), uniform division officer

"A federal air marshal offers a guide to observing and evaluating your surroundings.

"Quesenberry's nonfiction debut draws on his nineteen years of experience as an air marshal, a job that gives him "a first-class ticket into the world of covert surveillance, surveillance detection, and self-defense." In hundreds of settings, he has been the person paid and expected to know what's going on and to anticipate and counter any potential dangers. By contrast, as he quite rightly points out, most people relax themselves into a false sense of security by thinking "nothing will ever happen here" or "that would never happen to me." But even the author's cursory listing of some of the twenty-first century's worst outbreaks of terrorist violence all over the world should make it clear to readers that they can no longer afford such attitudes—they must take a large part of their safety into their own hands. Quesenberry's aim in his book is not only to change those attitudes, but also to arm readers with the basic perception shifts that will help them guard their own well-being. The foremost of these is "situational awareness," which the author describes as "the ability to identify and process environmental cues to accurately predict the actions of others." The adverb is crucial: readers are gently admonished to discard their reflexive prejudices and assumptions and "identify and process" what they're actually seeing in any environment (as the author points out, preset perceptions can sometimes blind a person to reality). In quick, sharply paced chapters full of well-chosen anecdotes and bulleted points, Quesenberry instructs readers on how to expand their awareness of the people and things in their immediate area, how to assume an aggressive mindset in order to anticipate how actual predators think, and even the basics of one-on-one self-defense. Much of what the author relates is elementary in nature—travel advisories all over the world urge some variation of situational awareness—but the clarity of this manual makes it stand out.

"A vigorous and memorable primer on heightening awareness to prevent or counter danger."

—KIRKUS REVIEWS

SPOTTING DANGER BEFORE IT SPOTS YOU

SPOTTING DANGER BEFORE IT SPOTS YOU

**Build situational awareness
to stay safe**

GARY QUESENBERRY
Federal Air Marshal

YMAA Publication Center
Wolfeboro, NH

YMAA Publication Center, Inc.
PO Box 480
Wolfeboro, New Hampshire 03894
1-800-669-8892•info@ymaa .com • www.ymaa.com

ISBN: 9781594397370 (print) • ISBN: 9781594397387 (ebook)

Managing Editor: Doran Hunter
Cover design: Axie Breen
This book typeset in Sabon and Midiet

20220105

Images by Shutterstock unless otherwise noted

Publisher's Cataloging in Publication

Names: Quesenberry, Gary, author.
Title: Spotting danger before it spots you : build situational awareness to stay safe /
    Gary Quesenberry.
Description: Wolfeboro, NH : YMAA Publication Center, [2020] | "Foreword by Lt.
    Col. Dave Grossman, US Army (ret.)"—Cover. | Includes bibliographical references
    and index. | Contents: Phase one. Understand the threat—Phase two. Build your
    situational awareness—Phase three. Develop personal defenses.
Identifiers: ISBN: 9781594397370 (print) | 9781594397387 (ebook) |
    LCCN: 2020932822
Subjects: LCSH: Situational awareness—Safety measures. | Safety education. |
    Self-defense. | Self- protective behavior. | Self-preservation. | Self-defense—Psychological
    aspects. | Instinct. | Crime prevention—Psychological aspects. | Victims of crimes—
    Psychology. | Violence—Prevention. | Women—Crimes against—Prevention. |
    Children—Crimes against—Prevention. | BISAC: SPORTS & RECREATION /
    Martial Arts. | SOCIAL SCIENCE / Violence in Society.
Classification: LCC: BF697.5.S45 Q47 2020 | DDC: 155.9/1—dc23

Note to Readers
Some identifying details have been changed to protect the privacy of individuals as well as the techniques and tactics employed by the Federal Air Marshal Service.

The authors and publisher of the material are NOT RESPONSIBLE in any manner whatsoever for any injury which may occur through reading or following the instructions in this manual.

The activities physical or otherwise, described in this manual may be too strenuous or dangerous for some people, and the reader(s) should consult a physician before engaging in them.

Warning: While self-defense is legal, fighting is illegal. If you don't know the difference you'll go to jail because you aren't defending yourself. You are fighting—or worse. Readers are encouraged to be aware of all appropriate local and national laws relating to self-defense, reasonable force, and the use of weaponry, and act in accordance with all applicable laws at all times. Understand that while legal definitions and interpretations are generally uniform, there are small—but very important—differences from state to state and even city to city. To stay out of jail, you need to know these differences. Neither the authors nor the publisher assumes any responsibility for the use or misuse of information contained in this book.

Nothing in this document constitutes a legal opinion nor should any of its contents be treated as such. While the authors believe that everything herein is accurate, any questions regarding specific self-defense situations, legal liability, and/or interpretation of federal, state, or local laws should always be addressed by an attorney at law.

When it comes to martial arts, self-defense, and related topics, no text, no matter how well written, can substitute for professional, hands-on instruction. **These materials should be used for academic study only.**

Printed in USA.

For my brothers and sisters in arms, both military and law enforcement. Your sacrifices will always encourage and inspire me. Keep fighting the good fight.

Contents

Acknowledgments   xvii
Foreword   xix
Introduction   xxiii

PHASE ONE——UNDERSTAND THE THREAT
Chapter 1 The Basics of Predatory Behavior   3
    1.1 How Predators Choose Their Targets—the Seven-Second PROD   7
    1.2 Perception   8
    1.3 Risk   10
    1.4 Observable Value   12
    1.5 Defenses   12
    1.6 Think Like a Predator   13
    Situational Awareness in Action: The Foiled Millennium Terror Plot   15
    Exercise: Target Selection   17
    Key Points   18

Chapter 2 Conducting a Self-Assessment   19
    2.1 Who Would Target You?   22
    2.2 What Would They Want?   25
    2.3 When Would They Strike?   26
    2.4 Where Would They Strike?   27
    2.5 Start Thinking Like a Protector   29
    Situational Awareness in Action: The Attempted Times Square Bombing   32
    Exercise: Using the Self-Assessment   33
    Key Points   34

PHASE TWO——BUILD YOUR SITUATIONAL AWARENESS
Chapter 3 The Basics of Awareness   39
    3.1 Defining the Threat—Perception vs. Reality   40
    3.2 The Levels of Awareness   42
    3.3 Understanding the Reactionary Gap   46
    Situational Awareness in Action: Joey Grundl's Big Delivery   48
    Exercise: The What-If Game   49
    Key Points   50

Chapter 4 The Next Level of Awareness—Comprehend, Identify,
    and Anticipate   53
    4.1 Comprehend the Situation: the Initial Scan   54
    4.2 Identify What's Important: the Detailed Scan   57
    4.3 Anticipate Outcomes   63
    4.4 The Role of Intuition   66
    Situational Awareness in Action: Ten-Year-Old Danny DiPietro   69
    Exercise: Environmental KIM's Games   70
    Key Points   72

PHASE THREE——DEVELOP PERSONAL DEFENSES
Chapter 5 What Comes Next   77
    5.1 Establishing a Basis for Action   78
    5.2 Avoidance—the Safest Option   80
    5.3 Escape   85
    5.4 De-escalation   87
    5.5 Confrontation   91
    Situational Awareness in Action: Lee Parker's Backpack   92
    Exercise: Route Planning   93
    Key Points   94

Chapter 6 Reinforcing Your Defenses   95
    6.1 Improving Mindset   96
    6.2 Minimizing Distractions   103
    6.3 Controlling Fear   105
    6.4 Building Confidence   113
    Situational Awareness in Action: Julianne Moore Stops a Kidnapper   117
    Exercise: Counting Drills   118
    Key Points   119

Chapter 7 Putting It All Together   121
    Situational Awareness in Action: Uber Hero Keith Avila   124
    Exercise: Six Steps to Spotting Trouble   126
    Key Points   127

Conclusion   129
Appendix: Self-Assessment   131
Bibliography   133
Index   137
About the Author   141

Acknowledgements

IT'S BEEN A LONG, winding road from the outset of this book to the actual finished product. At no point did I have a "eureka moment" when thoughts and feelings flowed directly from my mind, through my fingertips, and onto the page. The contents of this book have taken a lifetime to compile, and I've had plenty of help along the way.

Thanks to David Ripianzi and Doran Hunter for having faith in me and helping me to make this book a reality. Your guidance has made me a better writer, and I'm very thankful for the opportunities you've given me.

Thanks to Maureen Sangiorgio for helping me get this whole process started.

Thank you to my parents, who instilled in me my work ethic, my will to succeed, and my capacity for compassion and understanding. In a life filled with violence and uncertainty, the things you taught me have kept me balanced and sane.

An enormous thank-you to my brother Steven Quesenberry; you stood with me through some of life's toughest battles. I'll be forever grateful I had you by my side.

Thank you to my children, Josh, Elda, and Emily, for their mostly willing participation in the countless hours of room clearing, knife drills, sneak attacks, and "what if" games. I hope you found something useful in the incessant ramblings of your old man.

Most importantly, thank you to my beautiful wife Kelly. Your support and encouragement during our crazy life together made me what I am, and I will be eternally thankful for your patience and understanding. Anything is possible as long as you are with me. I love you!

Foreword

YOU HOLD IN YOUR HANDS AN AMAZING BOOK, unlike any other on the subject.

Many good books have been written about the critically important topic of detecting danger and protecting yourself and your loved ones from violence, books like Patrick Van Horne and Jason Riley's *Left of Bang* and Gavin de Becker's *The Gift of Fear*. Gary Quesenberry has integrated the best of such leading works with his own world-class expertise to create a uniquely useful resource. A work that is greater than the sum of its parts, and unlike anything else available on this critical topic.

This book also stands out because of Gary's incredibly thorough and comprehensive presentation of the main subject of this book: the art of *situational awareness*, a life-saving ability to spot danger in order to protect ourselves and our loved ones. The many case studies, drills, and exercises provided in this book will help to ensure mastery of this vital survival skill. I have read many books on the subject, and I can honestly say that no one has even come close to matching *Spotting Danger Before It Spots You* when it comes to teaching situational awareness.

This fundamental skill is key to surviving and overcoming the array of threats that confront the average citizen in the world today.

Finally, Gary Quesenberry is uniquely qualified to write this book. As a US federal air marshal, Gary lived and breathed situational awareness as an essential part of his daily life for decades. He has been there and done that. Gary's knowledge has been, as he puts it, "forged in the fires of real-world experiences." And he now passes that knowledge on to you in a powerful, masterful, and entertaining way, as all great teachers do. With all my heart I encourage you to study and apply the knowledge and techniques in this book to your own life.

As we love our families, as we love our nation, as we love our way of life, we must all rise to the challenges of the age. Armed with the skills taught in this book, you will not need to live in fear; you will live instead in a state of awareness and readiness. You will truly be "spotting danger before it spots you."

Dave Grossman
Lt. Colonel, US Army (ret.)
Author of *On Killing, On Combat,* and *Assassination Generation*
Director, Killology Research Group, www.killology.com

Lt. Col. Dave Grossman is a former West Point psychology professor, professor of military science, and an Army Ranger Lt. Col. Grossman's work has been translated into many languages, and his books are required or recommended reading in colleges, military academies, and police academies around the world, including the US Marine Corps Commandant's reading list and the FBI Academy reading list. His research was cited by the president of the United States in a national address after the Littleton, Colorado, school massacre, and he has testified before the US senate, the US congress, and numerous state legislatures. He has served as an expert witness and consultant in state and Federal courts, including *United States v. Timothy McVeigh.*

He helped train mental health professionals after the Jonesboro school massacre, and he was also involved in counseling or court cases in the aftermath of the Paducah, Springfield, and Littleton school shootings. He has been called upon to write the entry "Aggression and Violence" in the *Oxford Companion to American Military History,* three entries in the *Academic Press Encyclopedia of Violence, Peace, and Conflict,* and has presented papers before the national conventions of the American Medical Association, the American Psychiatric Association, the American Psychological Association, and the American Academy of Pediatrics. In addition, he has written extensively on the current threat situation, with articles published in the *Harvard Journal of Law and Public Policy* and many leading law enforcement journals.

Introduction

"If, then, I were asked for the most important advice I could give, that which I consider to be the most useful to the men of our century, I would simply say: in the name of God, stop a moment, cease your work, look around you."

—LEO TOLSTOY

I AM A FEDERAL AIR MARSHAL. That's the career path I chose, and for the past nineteen years, I've had a first-class ticket into the world of covert surveillance, surveillance detection, and self-defense. If I had to assess all the training I've received throughout my career and pick one essential skill I could pass along to everyone I care about, it would be situational awareness. Why awareness? Shouldn't it be something along the lines of precision marksmanship skills, or some high-speed, quick-finish self-defense technique? No. The bottom line is you can never fight what you can't see coming. For that reason, being mindful of your surroundings and capable of using what you see to accurately predict the actions of others are crucial skills when it comes to guaranteeing your personal safety.

When people think of situational awareness, they usually relate it to some spy movie they've seen. I always think back to a scene from *The Bourne Identity*. If you've seen the movie, you'll know exactly what I'm talking about, but if you haven't, here's a quick summary. The captain of a fishing boat finds Jason Bourne floating in the ocean. He has a bullet hole in his back, a mysterious bank account number embedded in his leg, and no recollection of who he is or how he got there. Although he has completely lost his memory and identity, he still possesses some pretty extraordinary abilities, two of which are some ninja-level self-defense skills and an almost superhuman capacity for situational awareness. In the scene I'm referring to, Bourne (who doesn't know that's his name yet) is sitting in a diner waiting for a female friend. When she comes in and sits down, they strike up a conversation about the best way for him to regain his memory. The woman tries to explain away Bourne's exceptional abilities, but he becomes frustrated and says, "I come in here and the first thing I'm doing is I'm catching the sidelines and looking for an exit . . . I can tell you the license plate numbers of all six cars outside. I can tell you that our waitress is left-handed and the guy sitting up at the counter weighs two hundred and fifteen pounds and knows how to handle himself. I know the best place to find a gun is in the gray truck outside . . . now, why would I know that?" I love that scene, but I think a lot of people have the misconception that that's how situational awareness actually works. Realistically it would be next to impossible to take all of that information in so quickly, but the good news is that these things aren't superpowers; they're basic skills we all possess, and once learned, they'll help you think more clearly and critically about your surroundings and how you interact with them.

My goal here is to take what's relevant in the world of situational awareness and personal safety and boil that information down to its simplest terms, which can then be easily implemented in your daily life. The techniques and exercises I'll have you practice work for everyone—parents, small children walking to school, teenagers going off to college, and whole families headed out on summer vacation. It works universally. When properly applied, this system of situational awareness will help improve your general understanding of how, when, and where violence occurs. It will also increase your chances of successfully detecting and avoiding danger no matter where in the world you may find yourself.

As a federal air marshal, my primary area of operation was Europe. At the time, there was a general feeling of unrest in that area that often turned violent. Knowing this, situational awareness played a central role in how I performed my job on the ground. Not every incident can be immediately identified and controlled, so it was essential to have specific skill sets that allowed me to spot potentially life-threatening situations before they occurred.

- March 2012: A gunman claiming links to al-Qaeda killed three Jewish schoolchildren, a rabbi, and three paratroopers in Toulouse, southern France.
- January 7, 2015: Two brothers stormed the Paris offices of *Charlie Hebdo* (a satirical newspaper) killing eleven people at the start of three days of terror. Another radicalized Muslim later shot and killed a policewoman before shooting more people at the Hyper Cacher market in Paris. The attackers were later killed in stand-offs with police.
- November 13, 2015: One hundred and thirty people are killed and hundreds wounded in a series of attacks by gunmen and suicide bombers at cafes, a rock concert, and a stadium in Paris. The Islamic State claimed responsibility.
- March 22, 2016: At least thirty-one people are killed and one hundred and fifty injured in three explosions at the Brussels airport and at a downtown metro stop.[1]

---

1. Belgium's federal prosecutor confirms that the incidents were suicide attacks.

- March 22, 2017: A man drove an SUV into a crowd on the sidewalk along the Westminster Bridge in London, killing at least four. After ramming the car into a barrier outside the House of Parliament, the driver exited the vehicle and stabbed a police officer to death before responding officers shot and killed him.
- June 3, 2017: Eight people were killed in two terror attacks in central London before police shot three suspects dead. The violence began when a van swerved into a large group of pedestrians on London Bridge. The suspects then jumped out of the van and proceeded on foot to nearby Borough Market, where witnesses say they produced knives and slashed indiscriminately at people in restaurants and bars. At least forty-eight people were injured and taken to hospitals, according to the London Ambulance Service.

These are just a handful of the attacks that happened during my time covering Europe, but they didn't "just happen." The attackers carefully surveyed and selected their targets. They made plans and conducted rehearsals. Unfortunately, some people have the mindset that "nothing will ever happen here" or "that would never happen to me." Air marshals don't have that luxury. We have to assume that every day could be the day and every place could be the place for the next attack. It's crucial you adopt that same attitude if you want to improve your situational awareness.

Before we begin, I think it's important to understand what you're up against when it comes to the frequency of violent encounters. The FBI's Uniform Crime Reporting (UCR) program describes violent crimes as those offenses that involve force or the threat of force such as murder and non-negligent manslaughter, rape, robbery, and aggravated assault. In 2017, there were an estimated 1.25 million violent crimes committed in the United States. That breaks down to an estimated 383 violent crimes per one hundred thousand inhabitants, or a little over two violent crimes committed per minute. Aggravated assault accounted for

65 percent of those crimes. Robbery took up 26 percent, rape 8 percent, and murder accounted for 1 percent. The report also shows that fire-arms were used in 73 percent of the nation's murders, 41 percent of robberies, and 26 percent of aggravated assaults.[2] According to data collected by the National Crime Survey and the Bureau of statistics, 73 percent of women and 89 percent of men will have been victimized by a violent crime in their lifetime.[3]

Given these statistics, I think it's safe to say that bad things happen and, unfortunately, bad things can happen to good people. We usually don't like to think about that fact because it makes us uncomfortable. Comfort is important to us, and we equate comfort with safety, but that way of thinking carries with it a fatal flaw. Turning a blind eye to the physical threats of the world so you can feel more secure is dangerous; it changes the way you act and carry yourself. It causes people to slip into patterns of behavior that are easily identifiable by criminals and, in their eyes, make you look like an easy target. It softens defenses, diminishes levels of awareness, and in the worst case, leaves you completely unprepared should you find yourself in a bad situation. Trust me, I'm speaking from personal experience.

Spotting Danger Before It Spots You—Build situational awareness to stay safe is broken down into three easy-to-follow phases:

1. Understand the threat.
2. Build your situational awareness.
3. Develop personal defenses.

Each phase will walk you through the various steps of developing awareness. At the end of each chapter you will find a refresher of the

---

2. Federal Bureau of Investigation, Uniform Crime Reporting Program, *Crime in the United States*, 2018 report, Fall 2019, 1–2.

3. Bureau of Justice Statistics, *Criminal Victimization, 2018*, by Rachel E. Morgan and Barbara A. Oudekerk, September 2019, 13.

key points as well as a practical exercise to help you put what you've learned into practice. I've also provided a self-assessment guide in the appendix to help you gain a clearer perspective on your current level of awareness and where you need to make improvements.

The methods I outline in this book were forged in the fires of real-world operations, and the lessons they carry were hard-won. The skills you take away from here can save your life if you are willing to put them into practice. There are no prerequisites; your past experiences may be very different than mine, but that doesn't mean you're any less capable of understanding your surroundings. You can be more alert, focused, and better prepared today than you were yesterday, so let's get started!

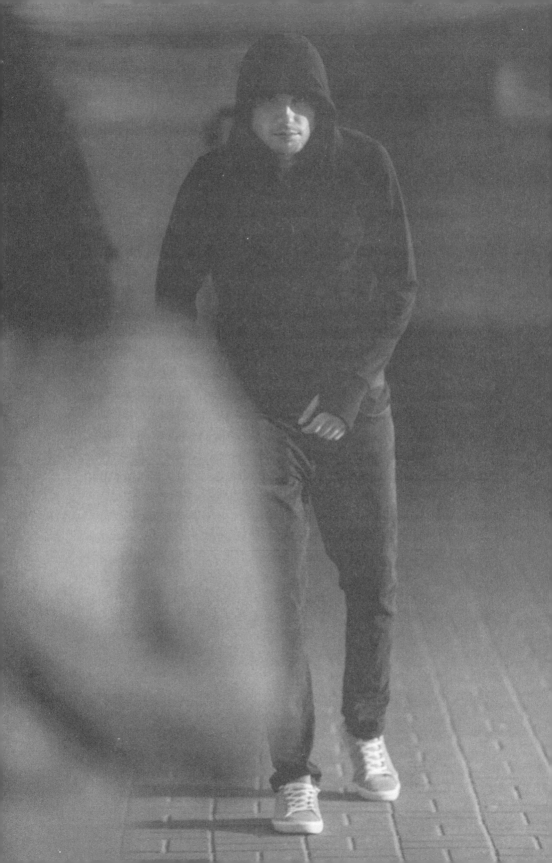

PHASE ONE——Understand the Threat

"I don't like that man. I must get to know him better."
—ABRAHAM LINCOLN

1

The Basics of Predatory Behavior

THE FEDERAL AIR MARSHAL SERVICE started out small back in 1961 with only a handful of agents. Back in those days, hijackings were fairly common. Between 1968 and 1972, there were 130 hijackings on American air carriers alone. The hijackers were typically driven by personal gain or just looking for safe passage to places they weren't supposed to go. They would demand that a flight take them to a place like Cuba and then ask for hundreds of thousands of dollars in ransom money before they would release the passengers. For years, airlines mostly gave in to these demands because they felt customers would find enhanced security at the airport more of an inconvenience than the possibility of a hijacking. Things changed significantly after four commercial aircraft were taken over by al-Qaeda terrorists and used as steerable weapons of mass destruction on September 11th, 2001. Now air marshals number in the thousands and serve on both domestic and international flights to detect, deter, and defeat acts of terrorism within the aviation domain.

As an agency, we thought we had a pretty good grasp of what the threat was, but in fact, we had become complacent. As we sat back waiting for the next cookie-cutter, standard-issue hijacking, the enemy was moving right under our noses, surveying targets and conducting dry runs for an attack we had never imagined. The signs were all there, but we missed them because we failed to give up on our old points of view.

Real situational awareness requires a shift in perspective. It's not enough to just walk around in a state of hypervigilance, thinking that nothing within your line of sight will go unnoticed. You have to be able to see yourself and others from the perspective of a predator. This isn't easy for a lot of people. For the most part, we all want to see the best in others, and the fact that someone else could possibly view us as a target of opportunity is hard to imagine. The unfortunate truth is that there are predators among us, and unless we can change the way we think, we may look like easy prey without even knowing it.

To better understand predatory behaviors, let's start by breaking down and categorizing the different types of predators and their basic motivations. In his book, *Facing Violence: Preparing for the Unexpected,* Sgt. Rory Miller breaks down predators into two groups: resource predators and process predators. A resource predator is looking for tangible items, be it cash, jewelry, or even your shoes. They've decided they need something and they're going to take it from you. Predators in this category include your basic mugger, pickpocket, or burglar. In some cases, if a resource predator confronts you and you just give them the thing they want, they go away.

Process predators, on the other hand, are much different. Process predators aren't interested in your watch or wallet; they get off on the act of violence itself. This category of predator includes the likes of rapists and murderers.

Motivations of the two categories of predators can vary, but violent behavior is primarily driven by one of four things: money, ego, territory, and emotion. Let's take a closer look at each.

1. **Money**: Like it or not, money is a consideration in almost every aspect of our lives. If you want a roof over your head, food in your stomach, and clothes on your back, you're going to need money,

plain and simple. Money is also a consistent factor in the commission of crimes. Some people have plenty of money, but they want more, and they'll do whatever it takes, legal or illegal, to get it. This is where you get your white-collar criminals who end up in jail for tax evasion, fraud, or embezzlement. In those cases, victims may have lost money, but they were seldom harmed physically. More commonly, it's the lack of money that drives people to commit irrational acts. Desperation can creep in, and people will go to any length to satisfy their needs. A friend of mine just sat as a juror on a capital murder case where a twenty-five-year-old man murdered his drug dealer over a forty-dollar debt. Most of us can't even fathom such an act over that amount of money, but money is just the beginning of the problem; the real issue starts when the need for money is fueled by addiction. According to the Bureau of Justice, more than 18 percent of inmates in federal prisons committed their crimes to get money for drugs. In addition, drug addicts committed 26 percent of violent crimes as defined by the UCR.[1] Alcohol, drugs, sex, you name it; if there's a need for it, you can guarantee that money is what gets it. For some people, when money is unavailable, crime is a reasonable alternative.

2. **Ego:** On the surface, this one seems to be a little less common, but we all have egos; it's the part of us that feels the need to be special. People will go to extremes to protect that feeling because it feeds their self-image, which can lead them into some pretty dangerous situations. We've all seen this play out either on television or in real life. Guy number one at the bar backs up and spills his drink on a lady's dress. The lady's boyfriend (guy number two) rushes to her defense and verbally attacks guy number one. Guy number one now has to save face in front of his friends and the other patrons of the bar, so he puffs out his chest and starts

---

1. Bureau of Justice Statistics, "Drugs and Crime Facts," https://www.bjs .gov/content/dcf/duc.cfm.

talking trash. Guy number two isn't about to back down in front of his girlfriend, so things escalate and become physical. Both guys end up bloody, broken, and kicked out on the street looking like fools. Overinflated egos often lead to bad decision-making. If you ever find yourself in a predicament where egos are taking over and it looks like confrontation is eminent, it's best to simply swallow your pride and remove yourself from the situation.

3. **Territory**: Humans are territorial creatures and will fight to protect what they consider to be theirs. An entirely peaceful, law-abiding citizen can become incredibly violent when they feel something within their territory has been threatened. A person's home is their territory. When a mother takes her children to the park, that area becomes an extension of her territory, and she will protect it viciously from anyone she feels poses a danger to her children. The same goes for criminals. They survey their surroundings and stake claims on everything from street corners to door stoops. They become aggressive and often violent when they feel their territory is being encroached upon. To avoid this, it's important that you become familiar with the places you frequent and be aware of any areas where your presence may cause problems.

4. **Emotion**: Violence is frequently driven by emotion. From jealous spouses to disgruntled employees and bullied teenagers, violent crimes such as mass shootings are often triggered by emotional responses. The level of emotion attached to religious beliefs has served as the primary influence behind acts of terrorism and the recruitment of others to extremist causes. Emotion is an incredibly powerful force, and it can be very unpredictable. Violence compelled by emotion tends to be excessively punishing.

Regardless of the motivating factors behind crime, the end result is always the same for the victim. The shock, emotional trauma, and physical damage suffered during an act of violence can resonate with victims for years. For this reason, it's crucial that you have a good idea as to why you may be targeted. The good news is that predators tend to stick to a specific set of conditions when selecting their targets. Knowing how they think and what they look for in a victim will be your first big step in achieving real situational awareness and go a long way in helping you to more accurately identify and correct your own vulnerabilities.

1.1 How Predators Choose Their Targets—the Seven-Second PROD

Just as criminals can be broken into two categories, criminals and terrorists alike tend to divide their victims into two groups: hard targets and soft targets. This concept applies to both people and places. A place can be considered a hard target when there are obvious countermeasures in place that would deter a possible attack, such as fences, cameras, and barriers that discourage unwanted entry. People can be considered hard targets when they appear aware of their surroundings, carry themselves with confidence, and look like they could handle themselves in a fight. Much like a bank, they are displaying visible defenses against an attack. On the other hand, places that are considered soft targets have no visible signs of security. There are no locks, cameras, or fences, and admittance is open and accessible to everyone. Similarly, people are soft targets when they display none of the outward signs of awareness or preparation. They look easy to approach and ill-prepared to defend themselves. Predators prefer soft targets because they pose the least amount of danger. They carefully measure risk versus reward and will almost always take the easier path. This process of elimination and target selection can be completed in as little as seven seconds. In that short period, a predator can accurately determine the following:

1. Their initial perception of who you are
2. The amount of risk you pose
3. Your observable value
4. Your visible defenses

These four factors, Perception, Risk, Observable Value, and Defenses, are what I refer to as the PROD. It's essential that you become familiar with them because when it comes to a violent encounter, they answer the question, "Why me?"

Ted Bundy was a serial killer in the 1970s who killed more than thirty women. Once he was finally caught, he sat for years on death row where he conducted nearly thirty hours of taped confessions. In these confessions, he laid out the types of women he targeted and the techniques he used to lure them in. At one point Bundy stated, "I can spot my victim by the tilt of her head as she walks." Since predators target those they perceive as weak, you must become the most unappealing target you can be. This all begins with proper situational awareness. Someone who carries themselves with confidence and purpose, who appears to be alert and aware of what's going on around them, will not be as appealing a target as someone who seems weak and oblivious.

Now that you know the basics of what predators look for in a target, let's start breaking down each element of the PROD.

1.2 Perception

How do you think other people view you? Do you come across as outgoing and independent, or are you more introverted and shy? How others perceive us has everything to do with the way we are treated, and it is a key element in how criminals target their victims. In 1981 there was a study conducted by sociologists Betty Grayson and Morris Stein that cast new light on how criminals picked their victims. Grayson and Stein hypothesized that potential victims were signaling their vulnerability to attackers through their gestures, posture, and exaggerated movements.

The researchers set up video cameras on a busy intersection in New York City and recorded people walking by between 10:00 a.m. and noon for three consecutive days. The tape was later shown to inmates who were incarcerated for violent offenses such as armed robbery, rape, and murder. The inmates were instructed to rate the people in the videos on a scale of one to ten, one being an easy target and ten being someone they would altogether avoid. When reviewing the results, two significant facts stood out.

1. There was a consensus about who would be easy to overpower and control. Every inmate chose the same people.
2. The choices were not solely based on gender, race, or age.

Grayson and Stein found that their hypothesis was correct and that criminals chose their victims based upon an entirely different set of standards than the ones they had previously assumed. Much like Ted Bundy, the inmates read the pedestrians' body language and used what they saw to make their choices. Basic movements the inmates identified as signals of weakness were:

- Short, shuffling strides when walking
- Not swinging their arms in proportion with their stride
- Exaggerated side-to-side movement when walking
- Head facing at a downward angle when walking

The inmates rated the pedestrians who had these traits between one and three, which identified them as weak and vulnerable. Pedestrians labeled a seven or above the inmates considered too much to handle in an altercation and were to be avoided altogether. They displayed the following characteristics:

- Medium to long stride when walking
- Arms swinging in proportion to their stride
- Body movement in vertical alignment, which was viewed as a strong and determined walking pattern
- Head level and eyes visible when walking

We may view ourselves one way but be seen in a completely different light by others based solely on our movements. Since you now know what physical actions signal vulnerability, you can take steps to protect yourself simply by modifying your body language. Just changing your posture and stride can make you look more like someone who would be difficult to subdue and who would likely put up a fight if attacked—in other words, a hard target.

1.3 Risk

Predators go through the process of target selection and attack planning to ensure success while minimizing risk to themselves. If they feel they can confront you with minimal danger, they are more likely to act. Some of the things criminals look for when measuring risk are simple enough. Are you with a group of friends? Do you look like the type of person who would fight back or cause a scene? Are you alert and moving with a purpose, or are you distracted? Some signals are more subtle; someone who frequently avoids eye contact, for instance, would be viewed as timid and therefore pose little or no risk to the attacker. That may seem inconsequential to you, but to a criminal, it could be the deciding factor.

Most criminals are looking for victims who will be easy to control. Sexual predators, in particular, look for people they can easily overpower as a means of avoiding risk. Todd Burke, a criminologist at Radford University in Virginia, says, "The rapist is going to go after somebody who's not paying attention, who looks like they're not going to put up a fight, who's in a location that's going to make this more convenient." In *Predators: Who They Are and How to Stop Them* by Gregory M. Cooper, Michael R. King, and Thomas McHoes, a convicted sex offender who raped seventy-five women across eleven states is quoted as saying, "If I had the slightest inkling that a woman wasn't someone I could easily handle, then I would pass right on by. Or if I thought I couldn't control the situation, then I wouldn't even mess with the house, much less attempt a rape there . . . Like, if they had a dog, then forget it. Even a small one makes too much noise. If I saw a pair of construction boots, for example, out on the porch or on the landing, I walked right on by. In fact, I think if women who live alone would put a pair of old construction boots or something that makes it look like a physically fit manly-type of guy lives with them out in front of their door, most rapists or even burglars wouldn't even think about trying to get into their home."

Risk or even the perception of risk is something that the majority of predators will go out of their way to avoid, so take a look at your current situation. What attributes do you possess that would pose a risk to predators? What areas of your life could you change to increase the risk level? Sometimes, little things can make a big difference. When you're out and about, just keeping your head up and looking around makes you more imposing. Walking with a dog is a fantastic deterrent. Traveling with a group or in well-lit areas decreases the likelihood you'll be targeted. The bottom line is this: anything you can do to increase the risk you pose to a predator will be worth the effort.

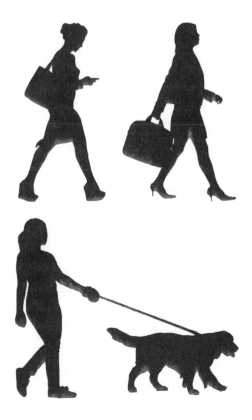

1.4 Observable Value

When you think of value, what comes to mind? A big house, nice car, and expensive jewelry? We all have an image in our mind of what real value looks like, but value is subjective, and it can look much different to you than it does to a potential attacker. The first thing you have to understand is that the one thing predators find most valuable is their own personal safety. It actually has nothing to do with the car you drive or the watch you're wearing. Criminals find those things attractive, but the real value lies in what they can take from you and get away with free from harm. That's why situational awareness is the number-one deterrent to street crime. If it even remotely looks like you'll see them coming, raise an alarm, or put up a fight to protect what's yours, predators will move along to the next target. That said, sometimes the level of value you display may be worth the added risk of arrest or injury. For example, if a criminal sees someone with an expensive laptop case slung over their shoulder, but they're in a more crowded area or with friends, the criminal may find the increased level of risk worth the reward of getting away with an expensive laptop computer. For that reason, it's important to be aware of how you appear to others. I'm not telling you what to wear out at night or what jewelry is most appropriate in public, but I will tell you that if you have anything of value on your person that's visible to others, it's a good idea to display more outward signs of security by moving with purpose, minimizing your distractions, and staying alert to your surroundings.

1.5 Defenses

Imagine for a moment you're a burglar casing two houses in a nice neighborhood. Both houses have well-manicured yards and give the impression that someone wealthy lives inside. You know you can find something of value in either house; the only question is which one to break into. According to a study conducted by the University of North Carolina at Charlotte's department of criminal justice and criminology, the majority of burglaries take place between the hours of 10:00 a.m. and 3:00 p.m. when most families are away at work or school. One of the first things you may do as a criminal is walk up to the house and ring the doorbell to make sure no one is at home. Let's say when you approach the first house you notice home security stickers on the front windows and door and the doorbell has a monitored security camera attached to it. You know right away you're being watched. When you ring the doorbell, you hear a very large dog barking on the other side of the entrance. Now a voice comes over an external intercom asking who you are and what you want. Seeing these visible defenses in action, you know that whatever of value may lie inside those walls isn't worth the risk to your personal safety, so you move on. At the next house, there are no security stickers and the doorbell is broken, so you knock; no dog is barking inside, so you move around to the back door. There are no signs of security, and the rear of the house isn't visible to any of the neighbors. You've found your target. The risk to you is minimal and whatever you may find inside will be of some value, so you break the lock and go to work.

This exact same concept applies to every person walking down the street. If someone is set on taking something from you, the first thing they will do is evaluate your visible defenses and decide on whether or not you have something of value or if you pose a threat to their personal safety. Regardless of the level of value you may possess, your defenses are what will serve as the deterrent to attack.

1.6 Think Like a Predator

When you try to see things from a predator's perspective, you have to flip switches in your mind that you may have never flipped before. You have to forget about social, moral, or religious norms and look at yourself and others as a predator would: a resource. You have to start looking past people's better natures and see their weaknesses. To get you in the right predatorial mindset, let's take a look at some commonly observed pedestrian behaviors. I'll list the behavior, and you determine if that behavior would make that person a hard target or a soft target.

1. A woman on the subway sleeping with her purse in the seat beside her.
2. A teenager standing in front of the mall waiting for his dad to pick him up. He is standing with a group of friends, his head is up, and he appears to be alert and undistracted.
3. A man walking along a crowded sidewalk. He is walking on the side closest to the doorways. He is wearing headphones and appears to be scrolling through social media on his cellphone.
4. A young woman is walking to her car from her office building. She has parked in the spot closest to the exit and under good lighting. She has her keys in her hand and is walking quickly while continually scanning her surroundings.

So how did you choose? If you chose subjects one and three as soft targets, you're absolutely right. Both of those people have something of observable value, their defenses are down, and the criminal's risk of getting caught or hurt during an attack is pretty low. The potential victims have put themselves in a situation where if they were approached, their responses would be strictly reactionary and driven by panic. The individuals in scenarios two and four, however, have made themselves more difficult to approach. They appear to be alert and aware of their surroundings, their defenses are up, and they look ready to respond quickly to any unwanted advances. This creates a problem for a potential attacker because it increases the risk of being caught or hurt during a confrontation.

There are no secret formulas or tricky algorithms here. As proven by the Grayson and Stein study, predators almost universally choose their victims based on their level of awareness and body language. The good news is that whatever you're doing now isn't set in stone; both of these factors can be analyzed and modified to improve your chances of completely avoiding a potential confrontation. But there's a process to conducting this self-assessment, which we'll cover in detail during the targeting exercise at the end of this chapter.

Situational Awareness in Action

The Foiled Millennium Terror Plot

On December 14, 1999, a twenty-three-year-old man named Ahmed Ressam packed his rented Chrysler sedan with explosives and drove onto the ferry from Victoria, Canada, to Port Angeles, Washington.[2] After clearing customs, Ressam planned on driving to Los Angeles where he would detonate a massive bomb outside the LAX airport on New Year's Day. At the Immigration and Naturalization Service inspection station in Victoria, Ressam presented agents with his Canadian passport. Ressam had torn the Afghanistan entry and exit stamps from his passport to avoid suspicion. The INS agent on duty ran the passport through a variety of databases and allowed Ressam to board the ferry. Later that day, Ressam arrived in Port Angeles in Washington State. He waited for all the other cars to depart the ferry, assuming that the last vehicle off would draw less scrutiny.

Alert customs officers assigned to the port began to notice that Ressam's behaviors didn't seem quite right. Despite the freezing temperatures, he drove with his window down, and he compulsively cleared his throat due to his prior exposure to the caustic chemicals used in making the explosives. He appeared to be overly nervous; he paced the dock of the ferry and was sweating profusely. These agents understood the baseline behaviors of the passengers that frequented the ferry, and Ressam's actions fell way outside of that baseline, so they quickly referred him to secondary inspection. When asked for additional

---

2. PBS, *Frontline*, "Ahmed Ressam's Millennium Plot," https://www.pbs .org/wgbh/pages/frontline/shows/trail/inside/cron.html.

identification, Ressam handed the customs agent a Costco membership card. As that agent began an initial pat-search, Ressam panicked and tried to run away but was quickly apprehended. Inspectors examining Ressam's rental car later found the explosives concealed in the spare tire well, but at first they assumed the white powder and gelatinous liquid were drug related until an inspector pried apart and identified one of the four timing devices concealed inside a black box. Ressam was placed under arrest, and thousands of lives were potentially saved due to the quick observations of the agents.

Whether it's a terrorist or a common street thug, those who wish to harm others typically go through the process of target selection and attack planning. Ahmed Ressam carefully planned his attack and chose his target based on the number of potential casualties a massive explosion would produce and the amount of media coverage it would receive. During the planning stages, Ressam chose what he felt was a "soft target" for his point of entry. He picked Port Angeles based on the amount of traffic it received daily and the limited number of staff working the port. He knew that if he timed his entry just right, the agents working the port would be nearing the end of their shift and more likely to overlook something during their inspections. What Ressam didn't account for during his risk-versus-reward assessment was the devastating effect one alert agent would have on his well-laid plans.

That's why situational awareness is so important. It's inevitable that at some point during the process of target selection, a criminal will reveal themselves through their own actions. These actions can only be observed and interpreted by those who are paying attention to what's happening around them.

Exercise

Target Selection

This is a great exercise to practice when you're out in crowded areas such as shopping malls, restaurants, or public parks. All you have to do is randomly pick someone out in a crowd. Using what you've learned in chapter one, evaluate them based on the PROD. You don't want to spend a lot of time staring at people; remember, this whole process should only take about seven seconds. Once you've picked someone out, follow the steps below until you've identified someone who lacks proper defenses and could be the potential target of an attack.

- **Step One: Perception**: Evaluate the person's body language, posture, and walking patterns to establish your initial perception of them. Do they appear to be unaware and timid, or confident and alert? If they are confident and alert, move on to another person in the crowd. If they appear to be unaware and timid, move on to step two.

- **Step Two: Risk**: Evaluate the risk involved. Does this person pose a risk to your safety? Do they look like they would put up a fight or raise an alarm if attacked? Are they with a group? If the answer to either of these questions was yes, move on to another person and start over. If the answers were no, move to step three.

- **Step Three: Observable Value**: Does this person have any observable signs of value such as a smart phone, backpack, laptop, headphones, expensive sunglasses, or purse? If they don't, move to another person and start over. If they do, move on to step four.

- **Step Four: Defenses**: Does this person display any visible signs of defenses? Do they look strong and capable? Are they alert to their surroundings and unlikely to allow an unwanted approach? If so, move on to another person and start over. If they display no outward signs of defenses, congratulations! You've found your target.

This is a simple observational exercise that increases your awareness of how others move through and interact with their environments. The more you practice it, the faster the process occurs and in time will take only a matter of seconds to conduct. By identifying those people who could be a potential victim, you also become more aware of your personal patterns of behavior and can more readily correct the weaknesses in your own defenses. Once you've got the hang of target selection, share what you've learned with friends or family members to make this a group exercise. The more knowledgeable those people are in terms of situational awareness, the more you increase your own personal defenses when you're out with that particular person or group.

Key Points
- Start looking at yourself and situations from the perspective of a predator.
- Understand the things that drive violence:
  1. Money
  2. Ego
  3. Territory
  4. Emotion
- Think like a predator (PROD):
  1. Perception: How do others view you?
  2. Risk: Do you pose a threat to possible attackers?
  3. Observable value: Are you displaying outward signs of value to others?
  4. Defenses: Are you displaying visible defenses against attack?

2

Conducting a Self-Assessment

NOW I'M GOING TO ASK YOU TO DO SOMETHING that may make you uncomfortable. I need you to take a long, honest look at yourself and evaluate what you see based upon what you've learned regarding the predatorial mindset. This exercise is known as a self-assessment and I've included a structured worksheet in the appendix to help you out with the process. Be honest about your current level of awareness and then use the PROD method to weigh out how others may perceive you, what risk you pose to potential criminals, your current level of observable value, and your personal defenses. Once that's established, we're going to break this whole process down and identify the four Ws, or the who, what, when, and where of a potential attack scenario. By uncovering your vulnerabilities, you'll have a pretty good idea of where your weak spots are and what steps you can take to minimize them. It's imperative that you conduct this evaluation, find those weaknesses, and make the appropriate corrections, but read through the whole book first. That way you have all the information you need before beginning the self-assessment. Trust me, you never want to put yourself in a position where you're being completely reactionary and making corrections only after the fact. Early in my career as a federal air marshal,

I was forced into a position where I had to completely reevaluate my own personal defenses. Unfortunately, this reevaluation was in reaction to what was regarded as the attempted abduction of my children.

It happened in 2003. I was assigned to the Las Vegas Field Office and primarily covered domestic flights along the Eastern Seaboard. My wife was a stay-at-home mom, and two of our three children were enrolled in the local elementary school. I was on an overnight trip to Baltimore when I got a call from my wife asking, "Did you try to take the kids out of school today? What the hell is going on?" I had no clue what she was talking about, but it was obvious she was distraught. After a few minutes of trying to calm her down, she explained what had happened. She and my youngest daughter (who was not of school age yet) had been out running errands. Instead of going home afterward, she decided to head to the school early and volunteer her time in the office, making copies for the teachers, something she did often. The staff at the school knew my wife well but didn't really know who I was or even what I looked like. When my wife showed up in the office, one of the secretaries made the comment that she was sorry to hear that we were removing our children from the school. Their belongings had been collected, and they were waiting in the counselor's office for their dad. My wife was obviously confused by this information, so the secretary went on to elaborate. A man identifying himself as Gary Quesenberry had called that morning and told the attendance officer he would be coming by the school and picking the kids up early. He said that because he worked for the government, he was being reassigned to a new office and the children would not be returning. The caller knew my name, the names of my children, and that I worked for the government. This information instantly sent my wife into a state of anger and confusion. It took several minutes to convince her that I was really in Baltimore and that I had not contacted the school. To me, this was a clear attempt by someone to get at my children. But who? What could I possibly have done to cause this? More importantly, how did I allow this to happen in the first place? I immediately called my supervisor and was on the next flight home. I had my wife make contact with the school resource officer and have law enforcement respond to the school. My supervisor, who was a former FBI agent, was on the line with my family walking them through everything that needed to be done. That was the longest flight I've ever taken.

In those early years of the Federal Air Marshal Service, several agents were targeted for attack by both criminal and terrorist elements, and we had been warned about the importance of protecting our identities and personal information. I thought I was fairly solid on these things, but obviously there were some gaps in my defenses. Looking back on this event I thank God that something moved my wife to show up at the school early. No one ever showed up at the school claiming to be Gary Quesenberry; perhaps whoever made the call saw the police presence and bailed out. There's really no way of knowing what would have happened if the guy would have shown up. We've always cautioned our children against strangers and how they should react if someone unfamiliar approached them. Hopefully, the school's system of identification would have eliminated any chance of someone removing the kids. I had no idea what had happened to cause this, but it was clear to me that changes had to be made. Those changes all started with a self-assessment.

Learning is a process that includes learning new things about yourself, and as you start on your self-assessment, you'll find that you identify and correct your weaknesses in four specific stages.

1. **Unconscious incompetence:** A person is unaware that a gap in knowledge exists. This is where people are utterly oblivious to the fact that they may be in danger. They are situationally unaware and when confronted with a problem have no idea how to react. This is what opens their eyes to the fact that corrections have to be made.

2. **Conscious incompetence**: A person becomes aware that a skill or knowledge gap exists and understands the importance of correcting those deficiencies. It's in this stage that changes can begin and it's why you picked up this book in the first place.

3. **Conscious competence**: A person understands how to use a skill or perform tasks like those you're learning here, but doing so requires practice, conscious thought, and hard work.

4. **Unconscious competence**: A person has enough experience with the skill that it can be performed without conscious thought. Situational awareness now becomes a natural part of their lifestyle and, because of that, a significant weakness in defenses has been corrected.

Regardless of what skill you are practicing, these stages of learning will always apply. Set your preconceived notions about security aside, and open your mind to new things. This is the absolute best way to ensure you're taking everything in and sufficiently developing your personal defenses. Once your assessment is complete and you've identified problem areas, you can begin implementing changes and putting your newfound knowledge to work.

2.1 Who Would Target You?

When the police showed up at our house to take a detailed report of what happened at the school, the first question they asked was about who would want to target us or our children.

"Is there an ex-spouse or stepparent who was still in the picture?"

"No."

"Is there an inmate from your past job as a correctional officer who may still hold a grudge against you?"

"Maybe."

"Have either of you made enemies since moving to Las Vegas?"

"No."

On and on it went, but we were never able to pinpoint a particular person who may have wanted to target my family or me. As you begin your self-assessment, you have to also start with the question, who would want to cause you loss or harm? A recent US Department of Justice report shows that the majority of violent crimes committed each year are committed by people the victim knew.[1] That means you are more likely to be attacked by someone you are familiar with than a perfect stranger. We all like to think we are a pretty good judge of character, but when it comes to protecting yourself and your loved ones, leave no stone unturned; everyone is worth a second look.

Here are some other statistics from the Department of Justice that may help to raise your awareness of who may consider you a target for attack:

- Among violent crimes, robbery was most likely to be committed by a stranger. Homicide was least likely.
- Seventy percent of violent crimes by strangers were committed against males. Seventy-seven percent of crimes by relatives were committed against females.
- Attacks by strangers are most likely to be carried out by more than one attacker, whereas single-person attackers are more likely to be someone known to the victim.

---

1. Bureau of Justice Statistics, "Violent Crime by Strangers and Nonstrangers," by A. D. Timrots and M. R, Rand, September 2019. This study concludes the following:
   - Persons in urban areas experienced higher rates of violent victimizations by strangers than persons in suburban and rural areas.
   - Strangers committed only 9 percent of violent crimes that occurred in the victim's home.
   - About half of violent victimizations committed by strangers occurred while the victims were away from home traveling, shopping, or engaging in leisure activities.
   - About 22 percent of victims of violence committed by strangers were injured, compared to 31 percent of victims who knew the offender.

Do not overlook the fact that there are evil people in this world. Frequently we see behaviors in others that we chose to ignore because we don't want to know the truth about their intentions; we want to believe that people are better than they are and that no one would ever have a reason to harm us. Unfortunately, we tend to look away even when the potential offender is someone close to us.

Jeffrey Dahmer was a notorious serial killer who murdered, raped, and dismembered seventeen young men between 1978 and 1991. Jeffrey's father, Lionel Dahmer, wrote a book about his son and his horrific crimes after Jeffrey's trial in 1992. Lionel realized that the way he'd interpreted Jeffrey's behaviors as a young man had been naïve. He essentially knew something was wrong with his son but looked the other way because he didn't want to believe what his senses were telling him. "I allowed myself to believe Jeff," Lionel stated, "to accept all his answers regardless of how implausible they might seem. . . . More than anything, I allowed myself to believe that there was a line in Jeff, a line he wouldn't cross . . . my life became an exercise in avoidance and denial." People are incredibly good at avoidance and denial. We choose to think that those around us have nothing but the best of intentions because that's the way we feel about ourselves. It's very important to open your eyes to the fact that bad people exist, and those people want to either take what you have or hurt you just for the hell of it. I realize you can't go through life thinking everyone is out to get you, but you have to acknowledge they are out there, and they're sizing you up.

As you begin your self-assessment, make a list of the people who may have grudges against you, or raise your suspicion for any reason. Have you made anyone angry lately? Have you severed ties with someone close to you who may still want your attention? Are there strangers in your life who repeatedly pop up in random places? Give it a lot of thought and make your list. This isn't necessarily a physical list of people you plan on systematically cutting out of your life; this is simply a mental exercise to help you work through the process of narrowing down potential threats to your personal safety. If you should choose to write them down, use the self-assessment guide in the appendix to help you organize your thoughts. That guy who got aggressive with you over a parking spot, he's on the list. The ex who keeps stalking you on social media, put him or her on the list. That stranger who shows up beside you every day at the subway station, he's definitely on the list. Revisit and update your list often, pay very close attention to your personal interactions with others, and make a note of any changes in attitude or behavior. This is another important step in raising your awareness level. If the same person repeatedly pops up on your list for separate reasons, then you should have your defenses up when that person is around you.

2.2 What Would They Want?

Next, you have to ask yourself, "What would someone want from me?" Resource predators see something you have, and they want it. Going back to the section on observable value, personal items such as watches, purses, backpacks, and clothing all hold some value to the resource predator, but in order to get at those items they have to go through a process of observation, decision making, and approach that can give them away well before they make their move. Process predators go through these same procedures, but they want nothing from you. It's the act itself that gives them what they need. It doesn't matter who you are or what you may have of value; their goal is to fulfill some personal desire that we may never understand. We'll get more into that later, but for now, it's essential to recognize that the things you carry with you can sometimes make you a target.

Now it's list time again. Start making a list of the things you have that a predator may find of value. Start with the everyday items you leave the house with: purses, briefcases, backpacks, jewelry, laptops, and similar items. Those all hold some sort of monetary value, but you carry them out into the world without ever giving them much thought. Now add to the list things you not only hold valuable but also consider priceless—your pets, your home, your family. In my case, someone had targeted my children. For whatever reason, they decided the value I saw in my family could be exploited to further their own needs. As we move through this process of developing awareness, you must note these things of value and see their possible significance from the perspective of the criminal. Only then can you begin to make plans to protect them.

2.3 When Would They Strike?

Given what you know about the who and what of a potential attack, when would be the best time for a predator to attack you? Take a look at your average week; at what points during that week are you most vulnerable? Is it when you're walking from your car to the office? Is it when you're alone on the bus or walking to school? Write those times down. All of them can be considered intervals of vulnerability, but there are steps you can take to ensure your defenses are up and visible.

The routine activities theory can help us better understand how our routines make us vulnerable to potential attacks. This theory is based on people's behavioral patterns and the situational factors surrounding crime. Basically, the routine activities theory states that a crime will occur when three conditions are met:

1. The presence of a potential and motivated offender
2. The presence of a vulnerable target
3. An absence of effective defenses capable of stopping an attack

The theory of routine activities gives us the perfect picture of when a violent attack would be possible. It's up to you to ensure that these three factors cannot be met. As we move forward, you'll begin to see that proper mindset and situational awareness are precisely what are needed to guarantee potential predators never have that perfect opportunity to attack you.

2.4 Where Would They Strike?

Look back at the times you listed as periods of vulnerability. For the purposes of this book, you are obviously the target, so based on the routine activities theory ask yourself the following questions:

- What are the chances of a motivated offender being in the area you are moving through?
- Do you have visible defenses in place to deter a possible attacker?

The higher the chances a potential attacker may be in the area, the more important it becomes to show the signs of alert readiness that turn predators away. Now I'm going to give you a fictional scenario. From the perspective of a predator, I want you to determine the best place to stage your attack. I know this type of roleplaying makes some people uncomfortable, but it's imperative that you be able to see things as a predator would so you can better identify and correct the flaws in your own defenses.

It's Friday night. You're a college student walking back to your dorm from an evening study session, so you're carrying your back-pack and laptop. Along your usual route, you spot a group of stu-dents who have obviously been drinking, and the situation ahead appears to be one of unruly misbehavior. This makes you nervous, so being careful not to make eye contact, you hesitantly decide to cut through a narrow passageway and avoid the rowdy group. The pas-sageway is dimly lit but cuts a little time off your route. As you approach the passageway, you decide to text your friends to let them know you're almost back to your room. Once on the other side, you cross a large, well-lit parking lot and proceed up the steps to your dorm room. Once safely inside you again text your friends to let them know you made it back.

Now let's take a look at our fictionalized student from a predatorial point of view and break this scenario down based on what we've learned so far. We'll do this using the PROD.

27

- **Perception:** Lack of eye contact, hesitation in movements, perceived as an easy target
- **Risk:** Walking alone, lack of confidence, visible level of distraction, poses little risk of being caught or hurt
- **Observable value:** Backpack, laptop
- **Defenses:** No visible signs of defenses

Based on these simple factors, a potential predator could very possibly decide to act against you. Remember, this only takes seven seconds to decide. Now, let's look at the four Ws: who, what, when, and where from the perspective of the student.

- **Who:** Is there someone near you or in the group of rowdy students who may have a reason to approach you?
- **What:** Are you in possession of anything that may be of value to someone else?
- **When:** Are there times you are vulnerable to attack?
- **Where:** Are there places or positions you've put yourself into that could possibly make you more vulnerable to attack?

Based on all these factors, what time did you pinpoint as being the best opportunity to stage an attack? If you chose the period of time inside the passageway when our student was on the cellphone, you're absolutely right. Now ask yourself, what are some steps the student could have taken to minimize the risk of being targeted?

- Have one or two friends from the study group walk back to the dorms with you.
- Keep your head up and proceed along your regular route in a confident manner.
- Place your laptop inside your backpack to lessen observable value.
- Minimize distractions by staying off your cellphone and alert to the situation in front of you.
- Don't let your perception of the group dictate your movements; make your decisions based on observable facts.

Much like our fictional student, by thinking through the seven-second PROD from the perspective of a predator and then asking yourself the questions of who would attack you, what would they want, and when and where would they strike, you will have a better understanding of your situation and make better decisions about your movements. All of this helps to effectively minimize the likelihood you are targeted for an attack.

2.5 Start Thinking Like a Protector

Now that we've conducted our self-assessments, it's time to flip the mindset switch from predator back to protector. I always considered myself a protector, but after the incident at my children's school, I had to take a long hard look at my defenses and completely reevaluate what it meant to provide real safety for my family. I realized I had fallen into the trap of believing I was impervious to attack based solely on my position as a federal air marshal. Complacency was my downfall, and the shock of the event led me to completely change the way I lived and communicated with my family. It was time to not only harden my defenses but also to pass along what I knew to my wife and children so their security didn't start and stop with me. Everyone had to get involved.

In December of 2007 a nineteen-year-old deranged killer entered the Westroads Mall in Omaha, Nebraska, and within six minutes killed eight people and wounded four others before killing himself. Back in 2007, well after the incident at the school, my three children were in their early teens, and like most families with teenagers, we spent a lot of time at the mall. Given what I knew about seemingly random acts of violence, I felt that it was necessary to inform my wife and children about the appropriate responses to situations like active shooter events. "If we're in the food court and gunfire erupts to the left, where do we go and what actions do we take?" "If we're entering a store and someone with a knife starts running toward us from the opposite end, what do we do?" The mental rehearsals provided by these what-if games were invaluable because they helped us to better prepare for situations we wouldn't normally dream of finding ourselves in. My children are all grown now, but to this day they'll tell you that the what-if games I played with them when they were young have helped them to be more aware and focused in their adult lives. Experts often remind us that "the body will not go where the mind has not been." Regularly asking yourself, "What would I do if . . . ?" and then visualizing your responses to those various situations, is an effective way to raise your level of awareness and decrease your chances of being caught off guard.

There's a great story about a man named James Nesmeth that revolves around the power of visualization and illustrates how effective it can be. James was an average golfer. He generally shot in the mid to low nineties but had aspirations of getting his game down into the low eighties. Unfortunately, his dreams of improving his golf game were interrupted by the war in Vietnam. There, Nesmeth was eventually captured and became a prisoner of war, where he spent seven years locked up in a four-foot by five-foot cell. To occupy his time and maintain his sanity, Nesmeth developed a mental routine in which he imagined playing eighteen holes of golf every day. Without the physical space to move within his cage, he would visualize every aspect of the game in his mind. He imagined what clothes he'd wear. He envisioned preparing his golf bag and loading his car for the drive to the course. When he was on the green, he could see every tree, hear their leaves rustling in the breeze, and imagine how the slight wind would affect the flight of his ball. He would then imagine gripping the club, setting his stance, and taking a few practice swings. Then James would step up to the ball and take his shot, seeing the ball float through the sky until it landed softly in the middle of the fairway. He thought through every step of his game in the greatest possible detail, never rushing and never skipping a step. From teeing off to sinking his putt, each shot was perfect, and every imagined movement was meticulous. He did this every day for seven years.

Eventually, James was released from prison and returned to his home in the United States. Shortly after his release, he decided to go and play a round of golf on his favorite local course. He shot a seventy-four that day, the best game he had ever played. Everyone was amazed that James knocked off over twenty points from his game without actually swinging a real golf club in more than seven years. James, however, knew the truth. He knew that the physical game was the easy part and the rigid discipline of his detailed mental rehearsals was where the progress really came from.

Australian physiologist Alan Richardson scientifically proved that visualization works when he had college students visualize certain athletic activities. He discovered that a person who consistently visualizes a particular physical skill develops "muscle memory," which helps them when they physically engage in the activity. Richardson chose three groups of students at random. It's important to note that none had ever practiced visualization techniques before the experiment. The first group physically practiced free throws every day for twenty days. The second group made free throws on the first day and the twentieth day with no practice in between. The third group made free throws on the first and twentieth day, but they also spent twenty minutes every day visualizing successfully making free throws. On the twentieth day, Richardson measured the percentage of improvement in each group. The group that practiced daily improved 24 percent. The second group, unsurprisingly, didn't improve at all. The third group, which had physically practiced the same amount as the second but added the visualization element, did 23 percent better, almost as well as the first group. That study can help us to understand better how visualization is essential when it comes to everyday tasks, but it is also an integral part of the what-if games I played with my family. By imagining various scenarios as we move through our environments and visualizing the possible outcomes, we better prepared ourselves to act should the need arise. Over time we all began seeing the benefits of these drills and how visualization significantly improved our level of awareness. It became our family mantra that it was better to prepare for violence and never face it than to be faced with violence and not be prepared for it. We had all learned that lesson the hard way.

Situational Awareness in Action
The Attempted Times Square Bombing

On a clear evening in May of 2010, a dark blue Nissan Pathfinder slowly pulled into a tourist-crowded block of Times Square in New York City near the entrance of the Minskoff Theatre.[2] The theatre was filled with visitors about to be released from a showing of the Broadway musical *The Lion King*. The driver of the SUV turned on the vehicle's hazard lights, exited the car while it was still running, and quickly left the area. These actions were so out of place in that part of the square that it quickly drew the attention of three alert street vendors. A T-shirt salesman named Lance, a handbag vendor named Duane, and a Senegalese immigrant named Alioune who sells photographs on the square all witnessed the actions at the same time and focused their attention on the abandoned vehicle. That's when they began to notice smoke coming from inside the car and what they believed to be the smell of gunpowder. All three quickly alerted police in the area. One officer approached the SUV and saw what appeared to be two large smoking canisters inside the vehicle. He immediately evacuated the area and notified the bomb disposal unit and local fire department. Upon arrival, the bomb disposal team used a remote-controlled robotic device to break out a window and explore the vehicle's contents. They found a triggering device made from two battery-operated travel alarm clocks connected by electrical wires to two five-gallon cans of gasoline, over forty M-88 firecrackers inside a twenty-ounce metal container,

---

2. Al Baker and William K. Rashbaum, "Police Find Car Bomb in Times Square," *New York Times*, May 1, 2010, https://www.nytimes.com/2010/05 /02/nyregion/02timessquare.html.

gunpowder, three full twenty-gallon propane tanks, and a metal gun locker that contained a pressure cooker stuffed with 250 pounds of urea-based fertilizer. Had this bomb exploded it would have sent massive amounts of shrapnel flying into the crowd killing hundreds, possibly thousands of innocent people. An investigation was launched, and within days a task force led by the FBI had zeroed in on the suspected terrorist, Faisal Shahzad, who was arrested trying to flee the country at JFK Airport. Shahzad, who was a naturalized US citizen from Pakistan, had also planned additional attacks on Grand Central Station and Rockefeller Center. Shahzad was convicted in October of 2010 and sentenced to life in prison without parole.

Needless to say, the actions of those street vendors saved countless lives that day. These weren't trained professionals like the agents in the story of the foiled millennium terror plot; they were the alert citizens of a city all too familiar with acts of violence. The events of 9/11 had forced them to conduct a deep self-assessment. They understood the ramifications of ignoring what was happening around them, and thanks to their increased level of awareness, they were all thinking like protectors.

Exercise

Using the Self-Assessment

Earlier in this chapter you were asked to conduct a self-assessment in the appendix of this book. Make it a habit to review and update these lists often, then evaluate your personal defenses based on the following:

- **Who:** Are you routinely exposed to the people you identified as someone who may want to hurt you? If so, try to minimize that contact as much as possible.
- **What:** When you find yourself in the vicinity of these people, are you in possession of something they may find valuable?

- **When**: Are there specific times during your daily routines you feel you may be vulnerable to attack?
- **Where**: Are there places or positions you've put yourself into that could possibly make you more vulnerable to attack?

Using these lists, continually identify the people, places, and circumstances that could pose a risk to your safety. When you find yourself exposed to one of these risks, make an effort to modify your body language and behavioral patterns to present a hard target to any potential attackers.

Key Points
- Conduct a self-assessment by asking yourself the following questions:
  1. Who: Is there someone near you who may have a reason to approach you?
  2. What: Are you in possession of anything that may be of value to someone else?
  3. When: Are their periods when you are vulnerable to attack?
  4. Where: Are there places or positions you've put yourself into that could make you more vulnerable to attack?

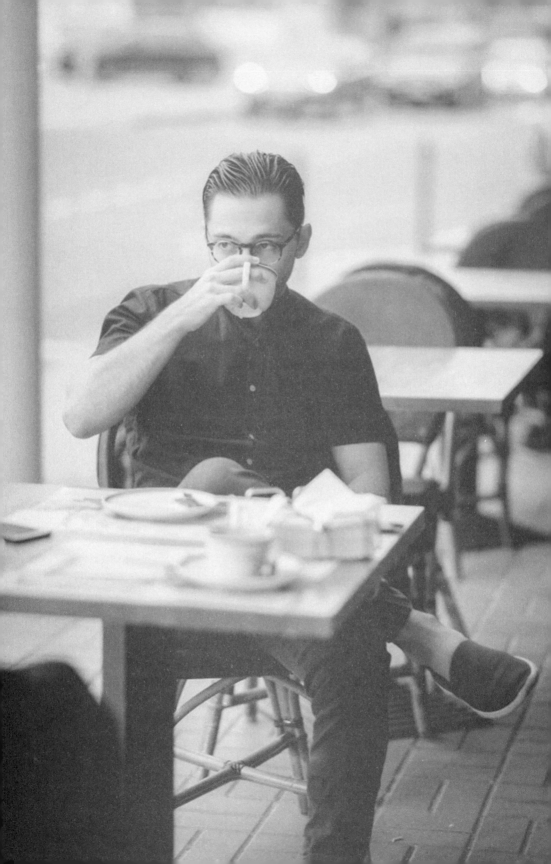

PHASE TWO—Build Your Situational Awareness

"You can observe a lot just by watching."
—YOGI BERRA

3

The Basics of Awareness

MY PERSONAL DEFINITION OF SITUATIONAL AWARENESS is this: the ability to identify and process environmental cues to accurately predict the actions of others. When most people think of situational awareness, they probably think of someone sitting with their back to the wall in a restaurant or constantly looking over their shoulder, but real situational awareness goes quite a bit deeper than that. It involves equal measures of comprehension, planning, and intuition. In some cases, when people set out on the path to become more of a hard target, they get their priorities backward. They'll get a concealed carry permit or pay lots of money for firearms training and self-defense classes, all of which are great, but those things apply to the reactionary aspects of personal safety. Real security starts in your own mind. The ability to logically process what's going on around you and spot danger before it has a chance to materialize should be your first priority. It allows you time to plan and act well before anyone else even knows what's going on.

Much like chess, there's nothing physical about developing your situational awareness; it's a completely mental game and requires focus as well as critical thinking. Lots of people imagine their lives like a chessboard. They have everything they need set up in a nice orderly fashion, and the threat only exists on the other side of the playing field, but after the first move, things become considerably more complicated. After both players make a move, there are roughly four hundred possible interchanges. After the second pair of turns, there are two hundred thousand possible move combinations, and after three moves, there are over one hundred and twenty million. Each turn requires you to dive deeper into the intentions of the other player, and each game evolves into one that has probably never been played before, each with a completely different outcome. Much like the beginnings of a violent encounter, it can be overwhelming. Now imagine being able to look at the board before all of that chaos and map out a solution that would always improve your chances to win. That is situational awareness: the ability to fully comprehend a situation before the first moves are made and plan your solutions well in advance.

Now that you have a pretty good handle on the concepts involved in the predatory mindset, which we covered in chapter one, it's time to move into the good stuff. But like any good training program, we're going to start with the basics. We're going to cover the various levels of awareness and how to remain observant without burning yourself out through hypervigilance. After that, we'll dive into the facts surrounding reaction times and how all of this factors into your personal safety; but first, I want you to have a firm understanding of how your perception of events can sometimes blind you to reality. One of the most important steps you can take toward hardening your personal defenses is putting aside what you think you know about the people who commit violence and focus on the things that define the reality of a situation.

3.1 Defining the Threat—Perception vs. Reality

It has often been argued that the world around us is subjective, that each individual's own perception dictates his or her reality. That would mean reality has to change from person to person. While it may be true that we all view the world differently based on our individual experiences, reality could not care less about your perceptions, and it does not adapt to your point of view. Reality is based on the cold hard facts that surround us, and unless you can sort fact from fiction, you may be putting yourself at a disadvantage. In the early days of the Federal Air Marshal Service, our reality revolved around the fact that hijackings rarely ended in death. It wasn't until after the events of 9/11 that we realized our view of the threat didn't match the reality, but by then it was too late. The rapid expansion of the service to meet this new threat was now completely reactionary.

Let's perform a little mental exercise. I want you to close your eyes and come up with a mental picture of what you think a terrorist looks like. Be honest with yourself; don't think about what's culturally or socially acceptable, just form the image in your head based on what you know about terrorism. What do you see? Where is this person from? What do they look like? Are they poor and underprivileged? Are they well off and nicely dressed? Come up with as much detail as you can. No matter what image you came up with in your head, I can guarantee the reality is much more diverse. Here are a few examples from just the last three years:

- October 1, 2017: A sixty-four-year-old white male opened fire on a crowd of concertgoers at an outdoor event on the Las Vegas strip in Nevada. Fifty-eight people were killed, and 851 were injured.
- October 31, 2018: A twenty-nine-year-old Middle Eastern male drove a rented truck into a crowd of joggers and bicyclists along a bike path in New York City. Eight people were killed, and twelve were injured.
- April 3, 2018: A thirty-eight-year-old female opened fire at the You-Tube headquarters in San Bruno, California. Three people were wounded.

- May 7, 2019: Two teenage students, one of whom was transgender, entered the STEM School of Douglas County, Colorado, and opened fire on their classmates killing one student and injuring eight others.

Now take your mental image of a terrorist and compare it to what we see in the real world. How does it match up? No matter what you may have envisioned, in reality, we have a sixty-four-year-old man with no apparent motive, a young female, one man from the Middle East, and a transgender teen. My point here is that there is no specific template for danger. It can come from anywhere at any time and be perpetrated by someone who before an actual attack was never even on your radar.

With all of these unknown variables, it would seem that just staying locked up inside your own home would be the safest option, but that isn't necessarily the case. The variables that affect your safety can be minimized by putting aside your preconceived notions and focusing specifically on actions. In the following sections, you're going to see that regardless of what form a predator may take, there are proven techniques that can be readily applied to help you identify the behaviors that accompany violent action. These "pre-incident indicators" can be applied universally regardless of race, religion, gender, or sexual orientation. They're identifiable patterns of behavior we all adhere to, and they dictate where your focus should be when you're dialing into your surroundings. We're going to take a much closer look at the details of human behavior, but let's first start with the most basic levels of situational awareness.

3.2 The Levels of Awareness

A critical element in your personal safety is learning about the various levels of situational awareness and how those levels affect your capacity to react. These levels of awareness are most commonly referred to as "Cooper's Colors," and they serve as the basis for the system of awareness you are about to learn. The Cooper color code system of awareness was developed by Marine Corps Lieutenant Colonel Jeff Cooper and includes five conditions, or colors, that represent a person's mental state during their daily activities. These five levels give us an overview of situational awareness and the psychological states associated with each level.

1. **Condition White:** In this condition, a person is entirely relaxed and unaware of what's going on around them. In the majority of cases, condition white is reserved for when you are asleep or when you find yourself in an environment you assume to be completely free of threats, like your own home. Criminals generally target people they deem to be in condition white. If you are ever attacked while in condition white, the chances of escape are diminished because your attacker caught you off guard. Your actions at that point will be completely reactionary.

2. **Condition Yellow:** This is a state of relaxed awareness. You appear to those around you to be entirely comfortable in your environment while paying close attention to the sights and sounds that surround you. This condition of awareness does not constitute a state of paranoia or hypervigilance. Instead, you've simply upped your awareness to a level that would prevent you from being caught off guard. Condition yellow is where you begin taking a mental inventory of your surroundings; you'll gauge your environment based on a preconceived baseline of behavior and start to look for people or actions that rise above that baseline. (We'll get more into that later.)

3. **Condition Orange:** At this stage, you have identified something that could be perceived as a threat, and you've narrowed your attention to that specific person or area. The transition from condition yellow to orange is subtle and happens several times a day

without you even knowing it. Think about driving to work. When you're driving, you're maintaining a consistent condition-yellow level of awareness (hopefully). Suddenly the car in front of you arouses your suspicion; maybe it looks like the driver is about to merge into your lane without checking his blind spot or signaling. You instantly notice this behavior and shift your level of awareness to orange to accommodate his actions. This is also the stage where you begin to put together spontaneous plans. Once the perceived threat has passed, it's easy to transition from condition orange back to yellow.

4. **Condition Red**: This is where you find yourself right before you act on your plans. In condition orange, you spotted a perceived threat and began the planning stages for an appropriate reaction. In condition red, the threat has materialized, and it's time to put those plans into action. This is where the heart rate becomes elevated, and the fight, flight, or freeze responses are triggered. Your body prepares itself for confrontation, and the adrenaline starts pumping into your system. Condition red is where your level of training has a significant impact on how the situation is resolved.

5. **Condition Black**: Condition black is much like condition white in that you do not want to find yourself there when the fight starts. Condition black is characterized by an excessively elevated heart rate (above 175 beats per minute) and a complete loss of cognitive ability. This is due to the lack of training necessary to properly deal with an active, violent threat. A person in condition black lacks the power to process the information being taken in effectively and becomes utterly useless in terms of response.

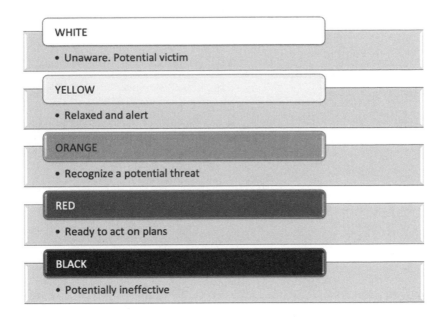

WHITE
- Unaware. Potential victim

YELLOW
- Relaxed and alert

ORANGE
- Recognize a potential threat

RED
- Ready to act on plans

BLACK
- Potentially ineffective

When it comes to maintaining proper situational awareness, condition yellow is where you want to be. You want to be in that casual, yet observant state that allows you to take in as much information as possible without completely stressing yourself out. That brings us to the next piece of the awareness puzzle, which requires planning. If you're in condition yellow and spot something you perceive as a possible threat, you have to start making plans for a reasonable response to that threat. This triggers what is known as the OODA loop.

Originally developed by Air Force fighter pilot John Boyd, the OODA loop is designed to help you quickly assess a situation and create a plan of action. The loop consists of four stages: Observe, Orient, Decide, and Act. Here's what happens in each stage:

1. **Observe:** You make an observation about something happening within your environment.
2. **Orient:** You understand environmental norms to help better identify potential problems.

3. **Decide:** You develop a plan of action based on information gathered during the orientation phase.

4. **Act:** You put that plan into action.

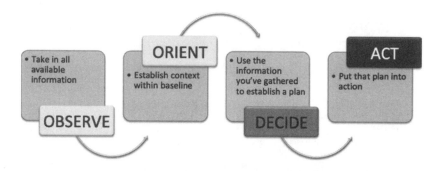

It's often said that action is quicker than reaction, but more accurately it's unanticipated action that catches you off guard and slows down your response time. By maintaining a condition-yellow level of awareness, you can more quickly identify possible issues and decrease your reaction times by being forewarned of a potential threat. Most often, the OODA loop process takes from one to three seconds to complete. This space of time is commonly referred to as the reactionary gap and can be decreased with proper training and practice.

3.3 Understanding the Reactionary Gap

There's a common misconception surrounding what's known as Hick's Law and the reactionary gap that I'd like to clear up. Hick's Law, named after British psychologist William Edmond Hick, describes the time it takes a person to make a decision as a result of the possible choices he or she has. Increasing the number of options also increases the time it takes to make a decision. In theory that makes perfect sense, but in practice, learning only one way to do a thing can get you hurt. Imagine getting physically attacked in a parking garage. Your attacker slams you against a car and takes a swing at your head. You've devoted your life to studying martial arts and Hick's law, so you know one perfect block to counter his punch to the head and you can perform it at lightning speed; the only problem is . . . that block didn't work. As the attacker swings again, you try the same block and still it fails. In reality, knowing more than one way to block a punch really doesn't slow you down that much. Let's say you know four solid blocks for a blow to the head. When you see that punch coming, deciding which of the four would be best at the moment takes only milliseconds. So if the first block doesn't work, you have several backups. Adding a fifth choice still wouldn't add any significant time, but it could significantly increase your chances of countering the attack.

In the Federal Air Marshal Service, we took a commonsense approach to self-defense. Instead of learning one way to block a punch or stop a knife attack, we would group our response techniques to accomplish a specific task within our counterattack. In the case of a knife attack, the first task was to trap the arm holding the knife. We had a few separate techniques we could use to accomplish that, but they all led to the completion of one task. After trapping the arm, we needed to "strip the knife" or knock it from the grasp of our opponent; again, there were several techniques we used to accomplish that. Then we would punch and kick like crazy until we created enough space to get to our gun. Once it's all put together, it looked like this:

1. Trap the arm.
2. Strip the knife.
3. Strike.
4. Create distance.
5. Go for your gun.

Five separate tasks but within those tasks were a number of individual options. By grouping your techniques, you can keep your responses logically organized, and if one fails, you still have a few reliable backups. When it comes to confrontation, you should divide your reactions into four categories: avoidance, escape and evasion, de-escalation, and confrontation. Each of the techniques you will learn in this book will fall into one of those four groups. Hick's Law is important to study, and the science behind it is valid, but don't trick yourself into thinking that it translates well to self-defense. Arm yourself with as many options as you can effectively practice, but remember to keep your techniques simple and to the point. Real violence doesn't look like it does in the movies. When confronted by an attacker, your goal isn't to go tit for tat with the guy in a dazzling array of punches and counterpunches. Your goal is purely survival and eventual escape. In almost every case, the best solution to the problem is also the simplest.

Situational Awareness in Action
Joey Grundl's Big Delivery

Joey Grundl was a Domino's delivery driver in Sheboygan County, Wisconsin.[1] One day during a routine delivery, Joey noticed something way out of the ordinary. As he was standing in the doorway taking a man's money and counting out change, he happened to look into the house and noticed a woman sitting on a couch in the background. In an attempt to communicate with the alert deliveryman, the woman pointed at her eye, which appeared to be bruised, and mouthed the words, "Help me." Not wanting to draw undue attention to the woman, Joey remained calm and tried to look distracted. After completing his transaction with the man and returning to his car, he immediately called 911. "I had a delivery. It was a middle-aged couple. The woman clearly had a black eye. She pointed to it, and I swear she mouthed, 'Help me,'" Joey had told the operator.

As it turned out, the man in the house was the woman's ex-boyfriend. He had forcefully entered her home and immediately became abusive. She tried to escape and got to her phone to call the police, but the man

---

1. Angel Torres, "Pizza Delivery Driver Helps Thwart Assault of Woman in Her Home, Police Say," NBC News, October 1, 2018, https://www.nbcnews.com/news/amp/ncna915546.

ripped the phone from her hand, punched her in the face, and dragged her upstairs where he tied her to the bed. The woman later told investigators he had shoved a towel in her mouth so "nobody would be able to hear her." For thirty minutes, the woman struggled to breathe and feared she was going to die. Eventually, the man untied her and brought her back downstairs where she creatively convinced him to order a pizza. That's when Joey showed up and took action. When police arrived, the woman called out for help, and the man was promptly arrested and charged with strangulation and suffocation, false imprisonment, battery, intimidation of a victim, and burglary. The woman told police that she "truly believed he was going to kill her that night. . . . I'm grateful that the delivery driver was paying attention because it could have been a lot worse."

When you dissect this scenario based on observation, orientation, decision-making, and action (the OODA loop), it's easy to see how calm planning and decisiveness can save lives. When Joey observed the woman sitting on the couch with a black eye, asking for help, he was thrown off guard and quickly had to orient himself to the situation. He knew that if he drew attention to the woman, he may have compromised her plan and put her in further danger, so he made the conscious decision to act distracted. He had decided before he ever left the door that something had to be done, so he made the plan to call 911. Once he was safely away from the scene, Joey acted on his plan, and within minutes the woman had been rescued from the situation. Joey Grundl is just another example of how average citizens can make a big impact when they exercise good situational awareness and sound decision-making.

Exercise

The What-If Game

What-if games are an extremely effective way to increase situational awareness and decrease reaction times in the event of a violent encounter. These games can be played in any environment and are most effective when you're playing with others. Here's how it's done.

Whenever you're out and about, whether on a shopping errand, picking the kids up from school, or out to dinner with the family, take note of your position within your environment and ask yourself questions about how you would react in certain situations. Start simply and then build on the scenario. You are only limited by your imagination. Here's an example.

The next time you're out to dinner with your friends or family think about this: what if someone enters through the back of the restaurant with a gun and begins shooting randomly? Ask yourself the following questions and determine the safest solution to the problem.

- Is there an exit nearby I can use to get everyone to safety? If people are flooding the exit, is there another avenue of escape? Identify as many as possible and mentally map out the best approach to each.
- Is there a place I can get everyone to that would provide appropriate cover or concealment? Identify as many as possible.
- If there is a break in the gunfire, is there something nearby I could use as an improvised weapon to subdue the shooter? If not, is there an opportunity to escape? How?

Remember that it's important to think through each scenario you come up with to the most desirable conclusion, which is to escape safely. These what-if games can help you mentally prepare for the unexpected and significantly decrease your reaction times should you find yourself confronted with violence.

Key Points
- Define the threat—know the difference between perception and reality.
- Understand the levels of awareness:
  1. Condition White: Relaxed and unaware of what's going on. If you are ever attacked while in condition white, the chances of

escape are diminished because your attacker will have been able to catch you off guard.

2. Condition Yellow: The preferable level of relaxed awareness. You appear to those around you to be entirely comfortable in your environment while paying close attention to the sights and sounds that surround you. You begin taking a mental inventory of your surroundings.

3. Condition Orange: A possible threat has been identified, and you've narrowed your attention to that specific person or area. This is also the stage where you began to put together spontaneous plans.

4. Condition Red: This is where you find yourself right before you act on your plans. In condition red, the threat has materialized, and it's time to put those plans into action. This is also where the fight, flight, or freeze responses are triggered.

5. Condition Black: Condition black is characterized by an excessively elevated heart rate (above 175 beats per minute) and a complete loss of cognitive ability. This is due to the lack of comprehension and training necessary to properly deal with an active, violent threat. A person in condition black lacks the power to process the information being taken in effectively and becomes utterly useless in terms of response.

• Continually assess your level of awareness and make sure you never slip into condition white when you're out in public. Strive to maintain a condition yellow state of awareness.

4

The Next Level
of Awareness—Comprehend,
Identify, and Anticipate

At this point, you have a decent understanding of the predatory mindset and how to use that knowledge to strengthen your own defenses. You also have an idea of how your preconceived notions about violent encounters can affect your level of awareness and diminish your likelihood of spotting the real threat when it shows up. Building on these fundamentals, it's now time to concentrate on the more focused aspects of awareness like comprehension, identification, and anticipation. These three elements will form the core of your awareness training and provide you with tools to accurately analyze your surroundings.

Since situational awareness is a mental exercise, I think it's only appropriate that, as with physical activity, we first warm up. A great way to do this is with what's known as a KIM's game, or Keep-in-Memory game. KIM's games are commonly used in military and law enforcement sniper training to increase observational skills. Candidates are given a number of random objects to memorize in a short period of time and then asked later in the day about what they saw. As the training progresses, the number of objects increases as does the amount of time between observation and questioning. This helps to build the candidate's level of awareness, attention to detail, and memory. Below, you'll find a picture of various items. I want you to study the image for thirty seconds. Memorize as much of what you see as possible, take in as much detail as you can, then without thinking about it, continue reading up to section 4.2. No cheating, and you only have thirty seconds. I'll ask questions about what you saw later.

KIM's Game

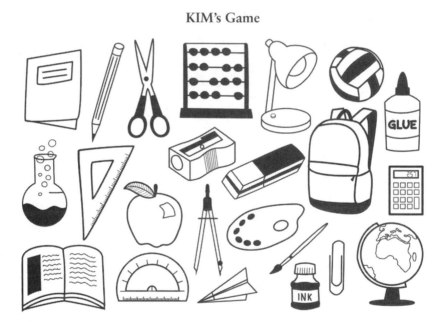

4.1 Comprehend the Situation: the Initial Scan

Whether we admit it or not, we are creatures of habit; we tend to live our lives within a specific set of patterns. We have a morning routine as we get ready for work, on the way to work we follow preexisting traffic patterns, and at work we know and understand the various moods and customs of our coworkers and how we should best interact with them. (Everyone knows not to talk to Brittany before she's had her tall non-fat latte with extra caramel drizzle.) Our entire universe moves based on predictable patterns. These patterns give us a sense of security, and when something changes and our patterns get modified, it affects us on an emotional and physical level; it tells us something is wrong. Think of these patterns that surround us as a baseline. These baselines can be applied to individual people, places, or situations. Every person has a different baseline of behavior. They can be talkative or shy, loud or animated; whatever set of behaviors is considered normal for that person is their baseline. They are both observable and predictable. Places have baselines as well; an airport, for instance, is expected to be busy and chaotic, full of travelers all moving to or from their respective gates with various amounts of luggage. Situations also have baselines; if you walked into a funeral, you'd expect to see a room full of somber, grieving people. You would expect it to be quiet with soft music in the background, and you would have a pretty good idea of how people in that situation should be dressed. As I said earlier, we live in a world full of patterns, and we all have a pretty good idea of what is considered normal in the areas we frequent. One of the most critical factors in good situational awareness is understanding these standard behaviors and being able to spot the things that fall outside of the established baseline. Being able to detect circumstances or actions outside of the baseline quickly is a process that starts with the initial scan.

Any time you walk into a space, be it a room, a parking lot, or a public park, you need to begin an analysis of the situation you're getting yourself into. You're not going to be sizing up potential opponents or memorizing license plates here; all you're doing at this point is asking yourself one question: "Does this place have a positive feeling or a negative feeling?" The only way to know the difference between the two is to understand what the baseline behaviors are. I'll give you an example from my days of working in a federal prison.

One of my favorite shifts to work in the prison system was "evening watch"; this was the 4:00 p.m. to midnight shift, and it was generally when all the action happened. I was scheduled to work one of the housing units. Each unit housed 128 inmates. When you walk into the unit on evening watch, the first thing you do is conduct a count of the inmates with the person you are relieving. Once the count checks out, and you know everyone is where they're supposed to be, the day watch officer goes home, and the inmates are released from their cells to roam the common areas until the main doors of the unit are opened for the evening meal. There are generally about thirty minutes between opening the cell doors and the unit being released. During that time, things can get pretty chaotic and loud. The TV rooms fill up and card games are started. Inmates rush to the laundry room or the showers, and there's a lot of movement and a lot of noise. That was the baseline for that cellblock. It was observable and predictable. One day when the cell doors were opened, something strange happened: there was very little noise, and there were only three inmates who chose to leave their cells and head to the TV room. It only took a few seconds to realize these behaviors were way outside the established baseline, and there was an instantaneous feeling of negativity inside the unit. It was obvious that something needed to be done, so I radioed for another officer to come over and give me a hand with things. We entered the TV room where the three inmates sat and began conducting pat searches. We discovered two "sissy shanks" (plastic toothbrush handles with razor blades melted into them); they probably won't kill anybody, but they make one hell of a mess. It turns out an inmate who frequented that TV room was behind on some gambling debts, and the three inmates were waiting for him to come in so they could cut him up. The other inmates had gotten wind of the plan and wanted nothing to do with it, so they all stayed in their cells after the count. Even the targeted inmate was aware of what was unfolding and very wisely chose to stay put.

Two things happened during that event that led to the discovery of the shanks and the plot to harm another inmate. There was an established baseline of behavior that everyone understood, and there was a set of actions that fell well outside of those observable, predictable patterns that were readily apparent during an initial scan. It's not exactly rocket science; you either get positive feelings or negative feelings about the places you go or the people you interact with. Some of what you feel will be based on intuition, and we'll cover that in more detail later. A few seconds of your time and a quick glance around can give you the first bit of information you need to determine whether or not an area, a person, or a situation is playing by the rules of the baseline.

Now the question presents itself, "What happens after the initial scan?" The answer depends on your findings. If the general feeling you get when you walk into an area is positive—for example, things are as they should be, people are acting the same way they usually do in that environment, and nothing really stands out as odd—then there really isn't very much to do from that point on. You can just continue about your business in condition yellow, frequently assessing your situation, and watching for any environmental or behavioral changes. That process of watching for changes is the beginning of what is known as a detailed scan.

4.2 Identify What's Important: the Detailed Scan

If the general feeling you get after your initial scan is a negative one, you have two options: leave the area immediately or start taking a closer look at your surroundings to gather more detailed information. What exactly aroused your suspicion and shifted you from condition yellow to condition orange? Was it a specific person, or an event within your environment that seemed outside the norm? Or was there a general shift in mood or attitude among a particular group? This is where the detailed scan comes into play. During the detailed scan, you're recognizing and collecting behavioral cues that help you to identify people within your area who may be up to no good. For instance, imagine you're at an outdoor beach concert in Southern California. Your initial scan revealed that all is as it should be—the mood is upbeat, the music is loud, and people are wearing the appropriate beach attire. You feel comfortable in these surroundings and everything seems to be well within the baseline. You are maintaining a condition-yellow state of awareness, so you're casually alert to changes in your environment when suddenly a guy walks into the crowd wearing a heavy winter jacket. This individual's behavior is obviously way outside the established baseline and could pose a serious threat to everyone's safety. But is the act of wearing a winter coat to a beach concert enough to warrant you tackling the guy to the ground or screaming "BOMB!" into the crowd? Absolutely not. So at this point there needs to be some corroborating information that justifies your suspicions before you can act. You need to quickly gather as much information as possible to make an informed decision as to an appropriate response. This process is called identifying baseline anomalies.

Federal air marshals deploy around the world and are exposed to a broad range of cultures. What's normal or acceptable in one culture may not be in another, so when you're performing a detailed scan of your area and looking for anomalies outside of your baseline, it's important to focus on those behaviors that are universal, applying to everyone regardless of age, race, sex, or background

Being aware of your environmental baseline and recognizing a potential threat early can save your life, but keep in mind that not all predators are large or overly aggressive, and not all are nervous or agitated; some are quite comfortable with committing acts of violence. They may not always be easy to spot or be overtly out of place. But predators do stick to particular types of actions that when identified early can alert you to danger before an actual attack can manifest itself. These behaviors are known as pre-incident indicators and commonly include the following:

- **Hidden hands:** The hands are what can kill you. Someone who is hiding their hands may also be concealing their intent to harm you.
- **Inexplicable presence:** Does the person who caught your attention have a reason for being where they are? Is their presence justified and their actions in alignment with the baseline behaviors of that area?

- **Target glancing:** Predators like to keep an eye on their prey, but in an attempt to avoid eye contact, they will continually glance at and away from their intended victim.
- **Sudden change of movement:** If you feel you are being followed and suddenly change your direction of travel, keep an eye on the people around you. If someone inexplicably changes their direction of travel to match yours, you could be their target.
- **Inappropriate clothing:** Like the man on the beach wearing a jacket, someone who is wearing more clothing than is appropriate may be trying to hide something.
- **Seeking a position of advantage:** Predators like to keep the upper hand. In an attempt to gain dominance, they will try to maneuver themselves into positions where they know they will have the tactical advantage. For example, an aggressor may try to back you into a corner where escape would be more difficult, or purposely block an exit.
- **Impeding your movement:** If someone inexplicably blocks your movement in a particular direction, there's a pretty good chance they're trying to funnel you into a position of disadvantage.
- **Unsolicited attempts at conversation:** If someone you are unfamiliar with approaches you and makes an attempt at unsolicited small talk, take a very close look at your situation. Are you in a position of disadvantage? Are there other people in the area? Has this person shown other pre-incident indicators that lead you to believe they have bad intentions? Attempts at small talk are often the predator's last move before the attack.

These are just a handful of known pre-incident indicators, but regardless of cultural differences, they're the common denominator when it comes to predatory behavior. One of these behaviors can be easily overlooked, and two may be coincidental, but once someone rises above the established baseline and has exhibited at least three abnormal behaviors, it's safe to assume action is warranted. In law enforcement this is known as the "Rule of Three" because it rises above the level of coincidence and into the realm of suspicious behavior. The action you choose to take may range from taking evasive maneuvers, alerting the crowd to the presence of a threat, or preparing for confrontation. If you see something that makes you uncomfortable, your best bet is to remove yourself from the situation and alert the police. If you choose to take action because all other options have been taken away from you, the potential threat must display the means, intent, and opportunity to harm you before defensive action is justified. We'll discuss each of those elements in greater detail later. For now, it's important to understand that the observed behaviors are just there to help you identify possible threats and articulate your actions to the proper authorities after the encounter.

Aside from the pre-incident indicators we just covered, there are also specific uncontrollable physiological reactions to stress that act as precursors to violent action. These are important to note because they hold true across all cultures, races, genders, and age groups. Here are a few of the more common physiological indicators.

- **Heavier than usual breathing:** When someone is under stress, his or her respiratory system is immediately affected. They begin to breathe more heavily or take sudden deep breaths to help distribute oxygen-rich blood to their extremities just in case they feel the need to fight or flee. Someone who intends to assault another person may appear to be breathing heavier than normal as they "psych themselves up" for the attack.
- **Appearing tense:** When we're placed under stress, our muscles naturally tense up to help protect us from injury and pain.
- **Posturing:** Frequently, people who feel threatened will naturally attempt to make themselves appear bigger. They'll puff out their chest, spread their arms, or become louder to ward off any potential threats or intimidate their intended victims.
- **Pupil dilation:** This is when a person's pupils appear larger and is often associated with fear and anger. Usually, a person's pupils are

two to five millimeters in diameter, but they can dilate to as large as nine millimeters when they feel threatened. This can take place within the space of a second and is a sure-fire way to gauge a person's emotional state—but it also requires you to be dangerously close to the subject.

- **Excessive sweating:** Sweating is a natural reaction to fear and stress regardless of the outside temperature. In late 2001, onboard American Airlines flight 63 from Paris to Miami, British terrorist Richard Reid attempted to detonate explosives he had concealed in his shoe. Reid's "shoe bomb" failed to detonate because sweat had soaked through his socks and into the explosive device. His actions drew the attention of other passengers onboard the flight, and they were able to subdue him until the flight could safely land. Reid was subsequently fined two million dollars and sentenced to three consecutive life sentences in prison.

These five items are not all-inclusive, but they offer a pretty good sample of normal physiological reactions to stressful circumstances. When paired with the known pre-incident indicators, they can quickly help identify someone who may be up to no good.

Since we're on the subject of identification, let's go back to our KIM's game. At the beginning of this chapter, you were given the task of memorizing as many objects as you could from the KIM's game photo. Without looking back at the picture, remember as much as you can about what you saw. I'll start off with a few simple questions:

1. How many items were there in the picture?
2. Did you see a book?
3. Were there any food items?
4. Were there scissors?
5. What number was on the calculator?

These are all reasonable questions based on the number of items in the picture, the time you were given to memorize them, and the amount of time that's passed since you first looked at the KIM's game. Most of what you saw should be easy enough to recall. Now let's go a little deeper into the detail.

1. What was in the small bottle?
2. Were the scissor blades pointed up or down?
3. What corner was the globe in?
4. What was between the scissors and the lamp?
5. Did the apple have a leaf on it?

As you can see, thirty seconds is sufficient to take in the big obvious items, but some of the smaller details can get overlooked when you don't have much time for close inspection. That's why it's essential to break your initial observations into the initial and detailed scans. The initial scan gives you a generalized idea of what's important while the detailed scan allows you to discard the irrelevant information and focus on the smaller things that can indicate potential danger.

KIM's games are a great way to improve memory and hone your observational skills. They're easy to set up or find on the Internet and the more you practice them, the better you'll get. In the Federal Air Marshal Service, we take the KIM's game concept and apply it to our environment.

1. What is the general mood?
2. How many people are there?
3. Is anyone in my area exhibiting pre-incident indicators?
4. How many exits are there, and which one is closest to me?
5. What objects in the area can be used as cover or concealment?
6. What items are available to help me create distance and escape?

This KIM's exercise can be adapted to any environment from walking around your neighborhood to driving in heavy traffic. You can walk into any room or down any street and treat it just like a game, plus it's a fantastic way to engage your children and begin building their observational skills as well.

4.3 Anticipate Outcomes

This is the heart and soul of situational awareness: learning to put aside your preconceived notions about what constitutes a danger and using what you've learned to accurately anticipate the actions of others. If you've been driving a car for any amount of time, you're probably good at this already. When on your morning commute, you naturally take visual cues from other drivers and use the information they provide to anticipate their actions. You can usually tell by the head movements of another driver if they plan on changing lanes even if they don't use their turn signal. On the flip side of that, someone may use their signal, but the absence of head movement tells you that they're about to come over into your lane without checking their blind spot. Having this information ahead of time allows you to correctly plan your responses and find the safest possible solution to the problem before it occurs.

Situational awareness is no different. The entire point is to use what you know about your surroundings to identify potential problems and plan appropriate responses should one of those problems materialize. If that happens, it's just a matter of picking the reaction that gives you the desired outcome. Here's an example. Mom sets three-year-old Johnny at the table for a snack. There's a glass of milk sitting at the edge of the table within Johnny's reach. Mom sees the potential for multiple outcomes, one of which is Johnny knocking the glass onto the floor, shattering the glass, and creating a much bigger problem. To avoid this, mom moves the glass of milk and replaces it with Johnny's plastic sippy-cup. Crisis averted, and everyone is happy. Mom understood her surroundings, observed a potential problem, anticipated outcomes, and took preemptive measures to avoid danger. It's that simple, but some obstacles can stand in the way of good decision-making:

- **Failure to monitor the baseline:** If you are not frequently checking the baseline, chances are you'll miss critical information. Any action that rises above the established baseline could be a precursor to danger, so it's imperative that you continuously monitor the baseline for changes.

- **Normalcy bias:** We're usually so preoccupied with keeping everything normal that we tend to believe things will always function the way they're supposed to. This creates a problem when it comes to predicting violent behavior because we can't predict what we believe will never happen. This is where the what-if games come in handy. By mentally playing out our reactions to violent scenarios, we break normalcy bias and open our minds to a much wider range of possible resolutions.

- **Focus lock:** This refers to a form of distraction so attractive that it concentrates all of your attention on that one thing, completely blocking all other input from your mind. The smartphone is the number-one culprit when it comes to focus lock. It completely draws attention away from your surroundings and instantly puts you in a position of disadvantage. If you need more proof just head over to YouTube and you can spend an entire evening watching videos of people texting and tripping over everything from park fountains to their pets.

By avoiding these three obstacles, we can better focus on what's important and use the information we're presented with to better predict the behaviors of those around us. This is going to require a little self-awareness. If you catch yourself ignoring the baseline or becoming focus locked on something that isn't important, stop, recalibrate to your surroundings, and continue to analyze your environment. Remember to continually play out your reactions to various what-if scenarios and follow them through to a desirable conclusion, such as a safe escape from the situation. Always see yourself succeeding. This is a critical skill, and it can only be improved through diligent practice.

The next time you're in your local department store use this what-if scenario as a way of putting everything together. You walk in and your initial perception of the situation is a positive one. People are moving about with full carts, browsing the isles, and acting the way you imagine people should act in a department store. Everything seems normal. As you move deeper into the store you notice that a man appears to be following you. This man isn't pushing a shopping cart. His hands are pushed deeply into his pockets and he appears to be watching your every move. To verify your suspicions, you weave through several isles unnecessarily. The man is still following you. How would you react? Here are a few options:

- One safe option would be to move toward a crowded part of the store where others are gathered. Remember, a criminal's main concern is their own safety and not getting caught. The presence of a crowd may cause him to panic and break contact. When you enter the store make note of where crowds are most likely to be gathered.
- Another option may be to seek assistance from a store employee or security. Know how the employees dress and where they can be found. Where is the customer service counter?
- You could abandon your cart and move toward the nearest exit. You know where the main entrance is, but have you identified any secondary exits such as fire exit doors that may also be alarmed?
- If no other options are available, you could turn and confront the person, "Are you following me?" Make it known that you will not be an easy mark and that you're willing to cause a scene.

These are all viable options, and your reactions will be based on your perception of the situation. But remember that not everyone is a criminal or out to get you. Paranoia comes across as fear, and fear makes you look like more of a soft target. Most people you come across during your day are perfectly normal, productive citizens just like you. Perhaps you dropped something in the parking lot and this man is trying to return it to you. Regardless of the man's intentions, it's important that you be confident and prepared to act should the need arise. Have a solid plan of action in mind at all times to ensure your own safety.

4.4 The Role of Intuition

Another factor in identifying baseline anomalies is good old-fashioned intuition. Although it is sometimes subconscious, your ability to read others plays a massive role in detecting danger. We start learning to read other people from the day we are born. We all know how to do it, but we very seldom have the depth of knowledge we need to describe how it happens. Oftentimes, we hear others say things like "out of the blue," "all of a sudden," or "out of nowhere." Some of the violence we see in this world we deem as "random" or "senseless," but the truth is that violence is neither of those things. In most cases, violence is predictable and avoidable if you know what to look for.

One of nature's greatest achievement is the human brain, and it works most efficiently when it feels that its host is in danger. What most people refer to as intuition is actually a cognitive process, and when we feel threatened, this cognitive process moves faster than we can control or perceive. We often second-guess our gut feelings because we put much more trust in a logical step-by-step approach to thinking. Some of the signals our brain sends us to warn of danger we disregard as trivial and unimportant because it's too hard for us to cognitively connect the dots between what we see and the risk that lies ahead. We owe it to ourselves to pay closer attention to these "gut feelings."

There's science behind your body's natural reactions to fear even if you haven't consciously registered the fact that you are afraid. Fear stimulates your brain and triggers a release of adrenaline and other stress hormones throughout your body. This rush of adrenaline is what causes your heart to race and your palms to sweat. It's also responsible for goose bumps, which are what make your hair stand on end. Goosebumps are the result of a reflex that causes the muscles attached to the base of each hair follicle to contract; these contractions force the hairs outward and make them feel as if they're "standing up." The adrenaline rush also causes the blood to rush from your limbs and into your core to protect the vital organs. This creates a tingling feeling in your extremities that most people refer to as "the chills." We often experience these subtle signals, but don't recognize them for what they are. Our brains have taken in information that it quickly registered as a threat and passed that information directly to our adrenal glands, completely bypassing rational thought. It's often well after an attack that a victim can look back and remember with some level of clarity what it was that actually alerted them to danger.

In his bestselling book *The Gift of Fear,* author Gavin De Becker tells the story of a woman named Kelly who was held in her own apartment and repeatedly raped for three hours before she managed to escape. It's a story of intuition and how subconsciously registered information can sometimes be the key to surviving a violent situation.

Kelly was returning to her apartment after shopping when she entered her building and noticed that the ground-floor security door had been left unlatched. Kelly thought nothing of it, believing that one of the neighbors had left it unlocked and latched the door behind her as she entered. As she climbed the four flights of steps to her apartment, one of her grocery bags ripped, and she spilled several cans of cat food onto the stairwell. That's when a kind young stranger approached her and offered to help. Kelly knew most of the people who lived in her building, but she didn't recognize the young man. At first, she refused his offer to help, but the young man insisted, and Kelly eventually relented and allowed the stranger to help her with a couple of bags. Kelly stated later that she was apprehensive about the man but couldn't put a finger on exactly why she felt that way; she even admitted to feeling guilty for having these negative thoughts about someone who to this point had given her no reason not to trust him. When they arrived at the door to Kelly's apartment, she thanked the man and attempted to take control of the grocery bags. The man insisted that he would help her into the apartment. He even said that if she was uncomfortable, they could leave the door open; he promised he would put the bags on the table and go. Kelly again gave in and let the man inside her apartment. That's when the nightmare began. Three hours later, after being repeatedly raped at gunpoint, Kelly lay on her bed in disbelief that she had allowed this stranger into her home.

That's when the man got up from the bed, closed the window, and got dressed. The stranger then promised Kelly he wouldn't hurt her; he was just going to go to the kitchen to get a glass of water, and then he'd leave. Kelly knew he was lying and that the only way to save her own life was to get out of the apartment. As the man walked down the hall, he stopped to turn up the radio. Kelly had wrapped herself in a sheet and followed quietly behind him. As he moved into the kitchen, she heard the man open a drawer and start rummaging through her silverware. That's when Kelly opened the door and rushed out of her apartment. She managed to make it into an apartment across the hall and ultimately to safety.

Kelly's story is utterly tragic and in no way her own fault, but there are valuable lessons to be learned here in terms of awareness. What signals were overlooked that could have prevented this tragic situation from ever happening? Let's take a closer look at what pre-incident indicators were missed and how Kelly's intuition played a significant role in her survival.

The first thing Kelly noticed was that the security door was unlatched. She explained this away by assuming her neighbors had inadvertently left it unlocked, but the information was subconsciously filed away and played a big part in the "bad feeling" she had about the situation later. Next, there was the inexplicable presence of someone she did not recognize as a tenant of the building. The stranger then made unsolicited attempts at conversation by offering to help Kelly with her bags. Once they were at Kelly's door, the stranger impeded her movement and sought a position of advantage by gaining access to the apartment. Aside from the unlatched security door, there are four obvious pre-incident indicators that Kelly was aware of, but was unable to make the connection between the actions of the stranger and the danger that lay ahead. In later interviews with Mr. De Becker, Kelly recounted how she had made her decision to escape. At the time of the incident, she didn't really know how to explain what drove her to get out, but she knew beyond a shadow of a doubt that the man intended to kill her. After she had had time to recover and look at the situation more objectively, she realized how her "intuitive" desire to get out of the apartment had really been brought about by a series of actions that her subconscious mind immediately recognized as danger. The stranger had shut the bedroom window and turned up the radio to drown out any noise from what he intended to do next. The unsolicited "promise" not to hurt her, when no such promise was asked for, was an attempt to pacify her. The rummaging through the silverware drawer had been him searching for a knife to finish what he had come to do all along. These split-second inputs were what set off Kelly's flight response and saved her life.

A basic understanding of situational awareness, predatory behaviors, and pre-incident indicators can absolutely save your life, but the importance of recognizing and properly interpreting intuitive thought cannot be overstated. It's your brain's way of bypassing the sometimes slow and cumbersome process of logical thinking. It tells you something is wrong right now and that you need to remove yourself from the situation. Listen to it when it speaks to you.

Situational Awareness in Action
Ten-Year-Old Danny DiPietro
Little Danny DiPietro is a ten-year-old from Howell, Michigan, and the locals are hailing him as a hero.[1] One Saturday evening in January, Danny and his father were headed home from hockey practice. As they drove along the snow- and ice-covered streets, young Danny was alert and paying attention. As they approached their house, Danny noticed that a neighbor's garage door was open and saw what appeared to be a dog standing outside. Given that temperatures had fallen below zero, Danny got the feeling that something wasn't right. Once they got home,

---

1. Danika Fears, "'He Wouldn't Give Up': Hero Boy Follows Hunch to Save Elderly Woman," *Today*, January 30, 2014, https://www.today.com/news/he-wouldnt-give-hero-boy-follows-hunch-save-elderly-woman-2D12018216.

Danny explained to his mother what he had seen and why he believed it was out of place. His mom explained to Danny that there was an extreme cold advisory in effect and that no one would leave a dog out in such weather. Never one to give up, Danny insisted that his mom investigate what was going on. Mom bundled up and headed to the neighbor's house. Sure enough, as she approached the open garage door, she noticed it wasn't a dog outside but their elderly neighbor sitting outside the garage waving frantically. The eighty-year-old neighbor had fallen on some ice outside her garage and had been lying on the ice for two hours, unable to get herself up. Danny's mom called 911 and covered the woman with some old blankets from the garage while they waited for the ambulance to arrive. Once safely at the hospital, the elderly lady was treated for a fractured hip. The ambulance driver commented that if it had not been for Danny's attention to detail, the woman would have most likely succumbed to the cold and died.

Young Danny deserves the title of hero. Had it not been for his level of attention and comprehension of the situation, a woman would probably have died that night. Danny doesn't possess any special skills or talents that set him apart from the rest of us; he simply had his head up and was paying attention to what was going on around him. Danny fully understood what was normal in his neighborhood, and to him the presence of an open garage door in such extreme cold fell way outside of the established baseline for that area and warranted further investigation. This story illustrates the fact that situational awareness isn't just something that's practiced by law enforcement and military types. It's a way of viewing and analyzing your surroundings that can be adopted and implemented by everyone, even a ten-year-old.

Exercise

Environmental KIM's Games

Take thirty seconds to study the following picture and then ask yourself the following questions.

- What seems to be happening in this scenario?
- Is there anyone in this picture who stands out?
- Why do they stand out?
- What are some possible outcomes?
- What corrections can be made to improve this person's situation?

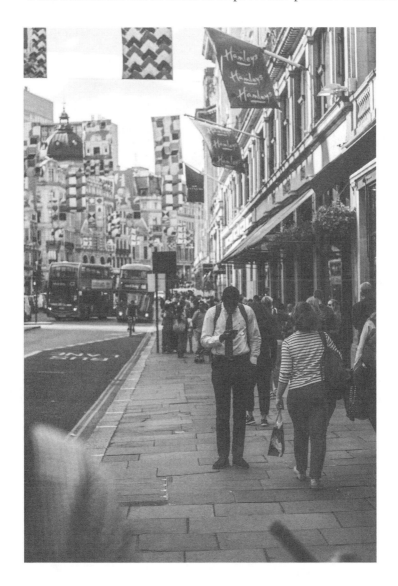

This is a basic example of baseline identification and can be applied to any environment. As I mentioned, if you have children, these environmental KIM's games are also a great way to get them engaged and started on the path to situational awareness. Here's what I use to do with my own children to make sure they were paying attention. The next time you're at the grocery store, or out for ice cream, wait until you're back in the car and then start asking questions about the people you interacted with.

- What color was the cashier's hair?
- Were they wearing a nametag?
- What was their name?
- Were they wearing glasses?
- Was there anything about this person that stood out?
- Did they appear to be happy? Angry? Sad?

Make it fun and offer rewards for correct answers. Teaching the importance of awareness at an early age can pay big dividends down the road when they become teenagers and start becoming more independent. If you don't have children, this is also a fun and productive exercise to conduct with friends or loved ones.

Key Points
- Comprehend the situation:
  1. Establish a baseline of behavior.
  2. Through observation, spot anomalies within the established baseline.
- Pay attention to intuition—if a situation feels wrong, get out of it.
- Spot the danger signs:
  1. Hidden hands
  2. Inexplicable presence
  3. Target glancing
  4. The sudden change of movement
  5. Inappropriate clothing

6. Seeking a position of advantage

7. Impeding your movement

8. Unsolicited attempts at conversation

- Physiological signs of danger:

   1. Heavier than usual breathing

   2. Appearing tense

   3. Pupil dilation

   4. Excessive sweating

- Things to avoid:

   1. Failure to monitor the baseline

   2. Normalcy bias

   3. Focus lock

- Find a way out: avoidance and escape are your two best options when it comes to personal safety.

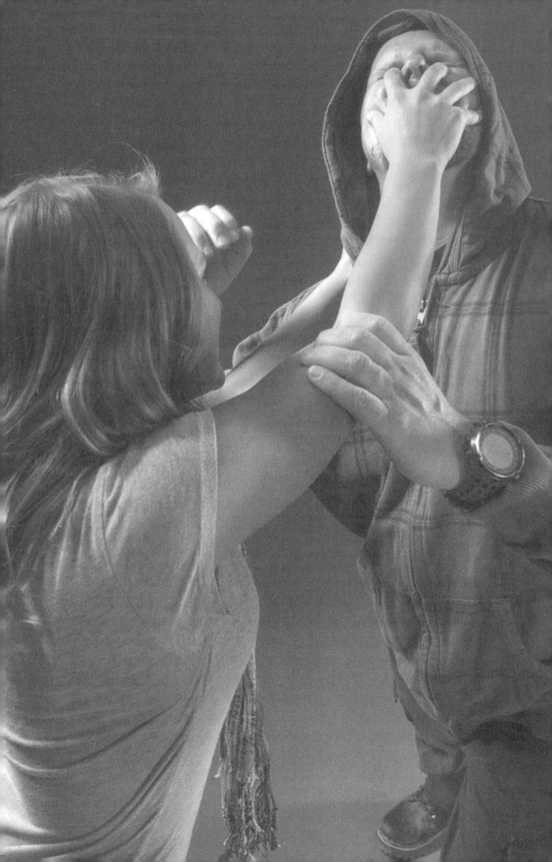

PHASE THREE—Develop Personal Defenses

"Self-defense is not just a set of techniques; it's a state of mind, and it begins with the belief that you are worth defending."
—RORION GRACIE

5

What Comes Next

NOW THAT YOU'RE FAMILIAR WITH THE BASICS OF AWARENESS, you can see that when it comes to the threat of a violent attack, being proactive is a much better option than being reactive. Knowing what to look for and how to interpret what you see gives you more time to develop a plan of action should the need arise. There are four basic options when it comes to self-preservation: avoidance, escape, de-escalation, and confrontation. Don't let the simplicity of these options fool you; people who are placed under enormous amounts of stress tend to overcomplicate things and in doing so can severely hinder their own chances of surviving an attack. When you're faced with a violent encounter, you have to approach the situation like you're solving any other problem.

- Identify the problem
- Determine your goals
- Assess the alternatives
- Choose a solution

This isn't always easy when you're not used to the devastation being caught off-guard can have on your decision-making process. That's why it's so important to use the what-if games to preplan your reaction to events before they happen. It keeps your solutions from getting overly complicated. Remember that when faced with a set of decisions, the best solution is usually the simplest one.

5.1 Establishing a Basis for Action

In their fantastic book *Left of Bang*, authors Patrick Van Horn and Jason A. Riley point out that people generally act within four specific groups of behaviors. They're dominant or submissive, comfortable or uncomfortable. Think about it this way. You take your significant other to the same restaurant every Tuesday night for dinner. When you walk in, you know the staff, you have a particular booth you like to sit in, and you know where the bathrooms are. To other patrons in the restaurant, you probably seem comfortable. Another customer walks in who's visibly upset and yelling. He's flailing his arms about and demanding to speak to a manager. This person's actions would fall under the category of dominant. In the corner, a waitress is chastising a busboy for not properly clearing the table. The busboy is obviously embarrassed and could probably be seen as submissive or uncomfortable. These are very basic behavioral categories, but they paint an accurate picture of how a person is feeling in a particular situation. When you walk into an environment and conduct your initial scan, you expect to see people acting in accordance with the norms. Aggressive is the norm for a mosh pit, but if someone were acting aggressively during a church service, you'd have reason to believe something was seriously wrong. It's when someone acts outside of those situational and behavioral standards that we need to start paying closer attention. To form a basis for action, you need to understand that just one unusual behavior isn't enough. That's why the Federal Air Marshal Service trains its agents to follow the Rule of Three we considered earlier: if you see three specific behaviors that fall outside of the behavioral norms, then you may want to start developing a plan.

Grouping three behaviors together that fall outside of the established baseline is the best way to predict someone's intentions, but it also helps to justify your actions should escape be impossible. The known pre-incident indicators and universal physiological reactions to stress listed in the previous chapter are all based on science and are easily articulable. One abnormal behavior may be written off as random or inconsequential, but if three of these behaviors are witnessed together, there may be a reason to reevaluate your need to be in that area.

If avoidance is impossible and you decide to defend yourself, there are three things you will need to consider when making the decision to act: does the person who poses a threat have the means, intent and opportunity to do you harm? These three elements will also be critical when it comes to explaining your actions to law enforcement should the event escalate to a use-of-force situation, so let's take a closer look at each.

1. **Means:** You have to ask yourself, "Does the person I perceive as a threat actually have the means to hurt me?" Most people have the means at some level: their fists, boots, or their size all serve as a means to do harm. Others may have visible weapons or at least indicate that they have weapons. After a violent encounter, you will be required to explain exactly what made you fear for your life. If you are claiming the threat was deadly, the means must be deadly as well.

2. **Intent:** To prove intent, you have to be able to show that the threat wanted to do you harm, and you must be able to articulate how you knew. A man screaming, "I'm going to beat the hell out of you!" is a pretty clear statement of intent, at least if his actions back up his words. If he then balls up his fist, aggressively moves toward you, and then draws his arm back to strike you, these are definitely corroborating actions to back up the statement of intent. Even if a person has the means to hurt you, and they've also displayed their intention to do harm, they still need the opportunity.

3. **Opportunity**: Intent and means do not matter if the threat doesn't have the direct opportunity to do you harm. If someone calls your home and tells you they have a knife and plan to come to your home next Tuesday to stab you, you can't legally take a pre-emptive trip to their house and kill them first. The threat has to be immediate.

If you've established that the potential threat has the means, the intent, and the opportunity to cause you immediate bodily harm or death, and you see a reasonable way to remove yourself from the situation, do it. It's that simple.

5.2 Avoidance—the Safest Option

The nature of self-defense is subjective. There is no one best way to defend yourself against an attacker, but in the majority of cases, if danger is spotted early and there is a reasonable avenue of avoidance, removing yourself from the situation gives you your best chance at survival. Even in the absence of obvious danger, there are several avoidance tactics that can go a long way in keeping yourself safe.

- Stay away from places you know to be high crime areas or frequented by dangerous people.
- Always be aware of your surroundings.
- Make yourself a hard target, or at least try not to look like a soft target.
- Do not provoke people or allow verbal conflicts to escalate.

Another effective way to avoid violence is simply to blend into your surroundings and become less visible to anyone who's seeking an easy target. In the Grayson and Stein experiment, the pedestrians who rated between four and six were completely ignored. Their "neutral" position in the crowd allowed them to move freely from place to place without being noticed at all. This neutral positioning is known as being "the gray man," and it's the next best thing to being completely invisible. There is security in anonymity, and that's why air marshals and intelligence operatives around the globe strive to be the gray man when moving through busy airports and crowded foreign streets.

There are plenty of situations you may find yourself in where you want to stand out in the crowd and be noticed. Maybe you're interviewing for a new job, and you're just one of many qualified candidates. Standing out and being memorable is definitely something that will help you out in that situation. You certainly don't want to be just one of the many talking heads that all blend together by the end of a long day of interviews. Your livelihood depends on you being memorable. Being original and noticeable is a natural instinct in humans. It's how we attract others. It's how authors get published, musicians get discovered, and it's how we find our partners in life. But in the world of predatory violence, being noticed can get you killed, especially if you're a noticeably soft target who's standing out in the crowd. When it comes to shielding yourself from violence, blending in is always a good option.

There are a lot of misconceptions about what it means to blend in with your surroundings. Blending in is not hiding. It doesn't involve sitting in the dark corners of a room with your face hidden behind a newspaper. Blending in requires you to be familiar with your surroundings and use what you know about your environment to mimic the look and mannerisms of the people who surround you. There are three primary aspects of blending in that you need to be familiar with if you're trying to vanish into the background.

1. **Clothing:** You always want to pick your clothing based on the environment, activity, and customs of the people around you. A three-piece suit may be appropriate when you're standing on the corner of Wall Street and Broadway in Manhattan, but wearing that same outfit while hanging out in the Englewood neighborhood of

Chicago may not be such a good idea.[1] Another thing to consider when choosing appropriate clothing is your destination. When you're traveling to an unfamiliar city or country, you really need to do your research and find out how the locals dress. One option is to pack light and buy your clothing from a local shop at your destination. I'm not talking about the t-shirt that says, "I went to Athens, and all I got was this lousy T-shirt." I'm talking about authentic native clothing that helps you to look like you belong there. Which brings me to my next point: identifying yourself as a tourist or even worse, an American tourist, can cause a lot of unwanted problems when you're in a foreign country. In Europe, Americans are sometimes viewed as uncultured and obnoxious, so go out of your way to adopt the tone and mannerisms of the locals in the area you're visiting. You should also limit observable value by not wearing unnecessary items such as flashy watches, expensive purses, or camera cases when you're traveling. These items always identify you as a person who may have money and can make you a pretty appealing target. When blending in, your best clothing options are always comfortable, durable, and inconspicuous. Keep it simple, no flashy colors or logos, and keep the color scheme muted and neutral.

2. **Body language:** When it comes to body language, confidence is king. Always look like you know what you're doing and where you're going even if you don't. At the same time, you don't want to appear overly confident to the point of seeming aggressive. This can make you stand out in the crowd just as quickly as being excessively timid. Move deliberately and with a purpose. When

---

1. In 2018 there were 675 homicides, 3,432 documented counts of assault, 1,843 counts of theft, and 344 counts of robbery in the Chicago neighborhood of Englewood. That equates to nearly one reported violent crime per hour in an area with a population of just 26,000 people. https://www.trulia.com/real _estate/englewood-chicago/2905/crime/

you're in a crowd of people, naturally there may be some interaction, so if someone approaches you, be friendly but cautious. Don't avoid eye contact or go out of your way to dodge conversation. If you'd rather be left alone and limit your interaction with others, there's plenty of ways to do that. When I'm working on the plane, I try to avoid conversation as much as possible with other passengers. My favorite technique for this is to just pop in a set of headphones and act like I can't hear anyone. You don't have to be listening to music, or even have them plugged in, but the act of appearing busy helps to limit the amount of interface you have with others.

3. **Positioning**: By positioning, I'm referring to where you sit, stand, or move within your environment. For instance, someone who looks for a quiet open corner in a cafe will naturally stand out more than someone who chooses to sit in the middle of the crowd. The same goes for movement. If you're positioned on the outskirts, you'll be noticed quicker than if you move within the crowd. When you isolate yourself, you become more vulnerable. If you don't believe me, just watch the Discovery Channel. Predators always hunt around the edges of a herd. I work and frequently move through airports and foreign countries. When I'm traveling, I always try to strike a balance between being on the edges and smack in the middle of a crowd. Suicide bombers typically try to make their way to the center of a crowd before detonating. This allows for maximum casualties and causes the most confusion. By positioning yourself between the outskirts of a room or group and the dead center, you're giving yourself a buffer from those direct-center attacks while maintaining your anonymity and proximity to possible escape routes.

Here are a couple of other handy tips I've picked up over the years to help you blend into your environment and avoid standing out unnecessarily:

1. **Know your routes:** Although you may be unfamiliar with the area, it's incredibly simple to consult a map and study the various routes to and from your destination. It's essential to do this ahead of time since continually consulting a map or your smartphone while en route to your objective will immediately peg you as a tourist and open you up to possible attack. Plus, having a good sense of where you're headed helps you to appear more sure of yourself.

2. **Keep close control of your money:** Don't flash your cash. When I was a young soldier stationed in California, I took a weekend trip to San Francisco with a few friends. I'm from Sylvatus, Virginia, so walking around in the big city sent my level of distraction off the charts. At one point, I split from the group and decided to walk back toward the hotel. I didn't know my way around the city, and since this was well before Google Maps, I got seriously off track. I soon decided I'd need to grab a cab to get back to the hotel, but I didn't know how much cash I had left. I pulled my wallet out of my pocket to see what was available. Before I knew it, I was laying flat on my back, and some fella was running away with my wallet. This guy had obviously been watching me for a while, just waiting for the right opportunity to strike. I gave chase for a couple of blocks but quickly realized I was being led further into a bad part of town. I had to set my ego aside and let it go. Fortunately, a wise old staff sergeant of mine had taught me to always keep extra cash in the bottom of my shoe for just such occasions, so I was able to catch my cab and make it safely back to my room. I had made several mistakes that night. I had split from the group, I was unfamiliar with my routes, I showed visible signs of distraction, and I openly displayed value. That was a hard lesson to learn, but from that moment forward, I knew the importance of keeping close control of my money.

   This rule also applies when you're traveling in a foreign country. Foreign currencies often confuse us. I can't count the number of times I've seen tourists in other parts of the world just hand a wad of bills to a cashier because they're unfamiliar with the local money system. Just like knowing your routes of travel, being familiar with the native currency helps you to appear more self-assured and decreases your chances of being targeted by a predator. Remember to always limit your observable value.

There are plenty of ways to keep from standing out or marking yourself as a soft target. The things I've listed above help, but the most important thing you can do to blend in with your surroundings is just to be yourself. Be polite to those around you and smile when it's warranted. You can't move through life constantly looking like a stone-faced killer; it's unnatural, and it's no way to blend in. Don't try to adopt some ridiculous disguise or alternative personality. Trying too hard is counterproductive and makes you look even more out of place. By just being yourself, you act more natural and confident, which makes you much less appealing to predators. More importantly, blending in and looking like a natural part of your environment also gives you a better vantage point from which to observe your surroundings. That's the end goal here: to be able to casually observe your environment and move from point A to point B, confident that you won't be caught off-guard and secure in the knowledge that you have a plan of avoidance should danger present itself.

5.3 Escape

In chapter four we covered the role of KIM's games in developing memory and how to apply those concepts to your environment. Taking note of exits, forms of cover and concealment, and even the presence of improvised weapons is useful information to have on hand when developing your plans. This is where all the information you take in regarding your surroundings will come into play and help you develop fast and efficient methods for escaping a violent encounter.

When it comes to escape, space is your best friend. If complete avoidance of a situation is impossible, distance removes the attacker's opportunity to do harm. It's unrealistic to assume you can keep a safe distance from everyone all the time, and this is where situational awareness aids in the process of elimination. If you're in an area you consider safe, and you're surrounded by people you know to be friends, then there's little need to concern yourself with personal space. If, however, you're in an unfamiliar setting populated by strangers, then maintaining a safe distance is prudent and can give you valuable time to spot and react to potential danger. Aside from keeping safe distances, several other options need to be considered when making an escape.

- Is there anything you can use to divert the attacker's attention from you?
- Is there any way to create an obstacle between you and the attacker?
- Were there any safe spaces you spotted along your route that you could retreat to?
- Are there any items nearby you can use against the attacker to create space?

These are just a few possibilities when it comes to making a getaway. Always remember that there is no substitute for sound awareness and planning. Know your surroundings and play out every conceivable scenario to a desirable conclusion, one where you end up safe and sound at the end. It may seem like a lot to consider, but the more you practice it, the easier it gets. Eventually, the whole process will feel completely intuitive.

5.4 De-escalation

In the absence of an escape route, de-escalation is the next best option. The quickest way to de-escalate a bad situation is just to give the attacker what they want, but keep in mind that this only works with a resource predator (someone who is using you to get something) and there's no guarantee of that. Process predators are a much different animal and could not care less about your material possessions; like the rapist in Kelly's story, they're in it for the crime itself, and you are merely a means to an end. The other option for de-escalation is through communication, but this can devolve quickly due to the overcharged emotional states that accompany confrontation, so it's important to be prepared should the situation change. Some key factors in effective communication are:

- Speak calmly but with confidence. Confidence is key here. Never let yourself appear timid when engaging a potential attacker in conversation.
- Try to keep a safe distance, but stay close enough to build rapport, or react if things turn bad—just out of hand's reach is a good rule to follow.
- Don't act scared. Acting scared or timid will only embolden an attacker and escalate the situation.
- Don't try to be intimidating. Trying to be overly intimidating toward potential attackers will only inflame their ego and escalate the situation.
- Watch body language—yours and the assailant's. Look for changes in posture and levels of aggression. Subtle changes in body language

such as balling up fists or slightly turning their feet to get into a "fighting stance" are good indicators that an attack is coming.

- Empathize—show some level of understanding of the attacker's situation. You may have to fake this part, but if it allows you or your family a safe means of escape, do it.
- Allow the attacker a way out. Never corner someone when you're trying to de-escalate a situation. Allowing the other person a way out gives them an option other than fighting.

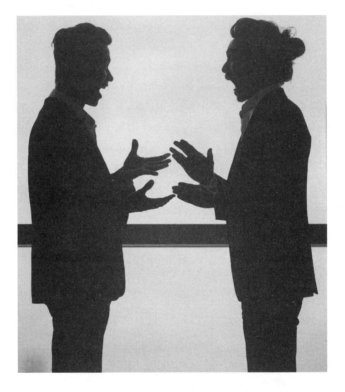

The what-if games I spoke of earlier were great when it came to opening my family's mind to the complexities of situational awareness. You can also take the games a step further and use physical roleplaying to get family members comfortable with using their communication skills.

My wife was always great at this, and to this day we all laugh about good ol' Mom walking into the kids' rooms and offering to sell them drugs. Any time this happens, the kids were instructed to yell, NO! BACK OFF! The mental image of my wife trying to sell imaginary narcotics to our children may be funny, but the lessons it taught were invaluable. They're good kids, and to this day, they've never been afraid to tell someone they don't know or trust to back off!

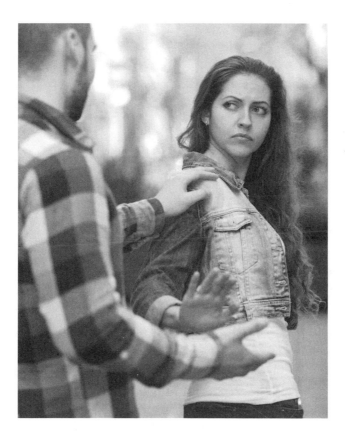

Back when I worked in the prison system there was a great book that we all passed around called *Verbal Judo: The Gentle Art of Persuasion* by the late George Thompson, Ph.D., founder of the Verbal Judo

Institute. His techniques for high-risk conversations when people are angry have been taught to police officers, military members, and security officers around the world for decades. Thompson's philosophy was that no matter who you had to deal with in stressful communication-based situations, certain universal concepts were always applicable:

- All people from all cultures want to be treated with dignity and respect.
- All people would rather be asked rather than told what to do.
- All people want to know why they are asked or told to do something.
- All people would rather have options as opposed to threats.
- All people want a second chance to make matters right.

He coined a reminder acronym for all types of verbal communication called LEAPS (Listen, Empathize, Ask, Paraphrase, Summarize), which is helpful in getting the other person to know that you are genuinely listening to them and not just waiting for him or her to stop talking.

- **Listen**: Be sure to make careful eye contact. Turn toward the other person, close the distance between you and them to build a sense of rapport, but leave enough room to react should the need arise.
- **Empathize**: Use validating statements with angry people such as, "I understand; I'm sorry that happened; let's figure out what we can do together to make this work; I can see you're upset; tell me what I can do."
- **Ask questions**: Ask open-ended questions, designed to get the angry person to tell their side of the story.
- **Paraphrase**: Accurately repeating what an angry or frustrated person has said to you can go a long way toward lowering the emotional climate by demonstrating that you really were listening.

- **Summarize:** Summarizing the conversation can help calm an angry person without ever saying the words, "Calm down."

When it comes to using effective communication for the purpose of de-escalating a heated argument, remembering these techniques will be your best bet and possibly the key to your survival.

5.5 Confrontation

I'm purposely keeping this section short. As I said in the beginning, the focus of this book is on situational awareness and ensuring your personal safety, but in the unfortunate event that avoidance is impossible, communication breaks down, and de-escalation is no longer an option, confrontation may be the only solution to the problem. This is a scary realization for a lot of people. That's why I recommend seeking out competent instruction in some form of martial art. There is no one best way to defend yourself in a fight, but whatever approach you choose to take, take it wholeheartedly.

In the movie *The Karate Kid,* Daniel visits the Cobra Kai gym where the sensei is preparing to drill his students. The pitiless sensei screams, "What do we study here?"

"The way of the fist, sir!"

"And what is that way?"

"Strike first, strike hard, no mercy, sir!"

Although the sensei and the students from Cobra Kai are the villains in the movie, I can't help but agree with their methods. When it comes to confrontation, speed, surprise, and aggression are the keys to survival. Once you've been backed into a corner and left with no visible means of escape, there's no point in waiting for the aggressor to attack. If the standards of means, intent, and opportunity have been met, then strike first and strike hard. Once you've created enough space to disengage, do so, and remove yourself from the situation as quickly as possible.

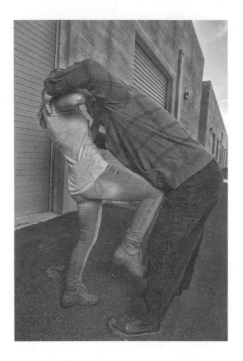

Situational Awareness in Action

Lee Parker's Backpack

Lee Parker was a homeless man who lived in Elizabeth, New Jersey.[2] At the time Mr. Parker had been carrying his belongings around in an old blue trash can, but because he had plans to attend a job fair, he decided that a backpack would be more appropriate. He and a friend began walking around town looking for anything that might suit his needs. That's when they stumbled upon what appeared to be a brand-new backpack lying on top of a garbage heap. At the time, it seemed entirely out of place but definitely warranted further investigation. When Lee

---

2. Colby Itkowitz, "Hailed a Hero, the Homeless Man Who Found New Jersey Bombs Gets Apartment, Job Prospects," *Washington Post*, September 24, 2016, https://www.washingtonpost.com/news/inspired-life/wp/2016/09/24/hailed -a-hero-the-homeless-man-who-found-new-jersey-bombs-gets-apartment-job -prospects/?noredirect=on.

realized it was indeed a brand-new backpack just lying there for the taking, he was thrilled and quickly grabbed it to see what was inside. Instead of the backpack being empty or full of old discarded items, Mr. Parker saw nothing but metal and wire. "I knew what I was looking at as soon as I saw it," his friend, Ivan White, later told news reporters. "It wasn't the cartoon bomb with the tick-tock, tick-tock, but it had wires."

Both men knew enough about what they were seeing to call the police immediately. Once law enforcement and the bomb squad arrived, it was determined that there were five separate bombs inside the backpack, which were believed to be connected to explosions the day before in New York City and Seaside, New Jersey. The bombs were safely detonated on-site by a bomb squad robot.

The locals in the area declared the two men heroes. "Hero? Nah, I won't go that far," Parker stated, adding that he was "just doing the right thing." Parker's friend, Mr. White, then told reporters, "I'm just glad I was able to realize what the situation was and react in such a way that, thank goodness, no one got hurt." Take a good look at that last quote. How does it align with the definition of situational awareness I gave you earlier? Pretty spot on, right? These men had no formal training; they just knew their area, spotted something outside of what they considered normal and, following a more detailed scan, realized that immediate law enforcement action was required. That's how this whole process of situational awareness should work, and just like Mr. White said, your goal should be to react in a way where no one gets hurt.

Exercise

Route Planning

Knowing your way to and from the locations you frequent is a basic skill, but make it a point to find as many different routes as possible and vary your travel patterns. This makes you less predictable and works whether you're walking, driving, or using public transportation. Here are a few things you can do when you're on foot to help raise your level of awareness, decrease reaction times, and improve your defensive posture.

- Keep your head up and continuously scan your environment for baseline anomalies.
- Don't approach corners too closely. Give yourself as much space as possible to help with visibility and increase reactionary times.
- Avoid unnecessary distractions.
- Keep an eye on people's hands.
- Pay close attention to the way you walk. Remember to stand up straight and move with purpose. Looking sure of yourself is a great way to deter potential attackers.

During your daily activities frequently reevaluate your posture and walking patterns. As this becomes more natural you can then add mental tasks such as target selection exercises and KIM's games to sharpen your senses and improve your overall awareness.

Key Points
- Establish a basis for action. Grouping three behaviors together that fall outside of the established baseline is the best way to predict someone's intentions.
- Before you act, ask yourself:
  1. Does this person have the means to hurt me?
  2. Has this person displayed their intent to hurt me?
  3. Does this person have the opportunity to hurt me?
- Know your options.
  1. Avoidance: The only way to ensure your safety 100 percent of the time.
  2. Escape: Know your exits and what's available to aid in your getting away.
  3. De-escalation: Use your communication skills to calm the situation.
  4. Confrontation: Always the riskiest option but sometimes necessary. If you have to fight, fight to win.

6

Reinforcing Your Defenses

WE'VE DISCUSSED THE DIFFERENCES between hard targets and soft targets. I'm sure by now you understand the importance of being aware and well prepared, but during your self-assessment, you may have spotted a few weak spots. Now we're going to cover ways to correct those weaknesses and reinforce your defenses. Regardless of how impenetrable you think your defenses are or how well thought out your plans for early detection and avoidance may be, there is always the possibility that something could slip through and catch you unaware. For this reason, it's crucial that you improve your mindset, learn to minimize distractions, control fear, and build confidence through practice and understanding. All of these things will help you to harden your defenses and round out your skill sets in the area of attack survival. They'll also change the way you carry yourself and how others view you, which will of course make you less appealing to potential criminals and help ensure your general safety.

6.1 Improving Mindset

Now that we've covered the concepts of predatory behavior and situational awareness, it's important to acknowledge that not every situation is avoidable. At some point in your life, you may find yourself confronted by something or someone you did not see coming. When this happens, you'll need to have a good understanding of what role your mindset plays in the outcome of those situations.

Every violent encounter consists of two separate battles: the one we fight in our minds before the confrontation, and the actual physical conflict. The doubt and insecurity that sometimes accompany confrontation can create a losing mindset and cause you to give up long before things turn physical. People often give up or lose their focus because they let those negative feelings creep in and take over. It's important to understand that people sometimes find themselves in horrible situations with little or no warning. If that happens you have to push negativity aside and focus on the best way to approach the problem. At this stage, it's more often than not the person's mindset that saves their life.

Take, for instance, Lt. Brian Murphy of the Oak Creek Wisconsin Police Department. Lt. Murphy was the supervisor on duty one Sunday morning in 2012 when he received the report of an active shooter in a nearby Sikh temple. Murphy quickly realized that he was closest to the scene, and within minutes he found himself face to face with the deranged shooter. Both Murphy and the gunman opened fire. Murphy's first shot missed, and he immediately began taking rounds. One round pierced Murphy's face; it struck his jawbone, went down his throat, ripped through this vocal cords and esophagus, and eventually bounced off his spine. He then took cover behind a car but said he realized immediately "it was a tactical mistake" because he lost sight of the shooter. The shooter then approached Murphy from behind and began to unload. One round struck Murphy's thumb, completely destroying it and knocking his gun from his hand. "About halfway through I'm thinking, 'When are you going to be done shooting me?'" Murphy said. Eventually one of the rounds pierced Murphy's skull. That's when backup arrived and began returning fire on the shooter, who at that point committed suicide. Fifteen rounds struck Lt. Murphy; three hit his ballistic vest, and twelve entered his body, but he was still breathing. What kept Murphy alive during that ordeal? He was admittedly frustrated with his own marksmanship and tactical decisions, so what kept him going? What kept him fighting back? Describing what was going on in his head as he tried to crawl away from his attacker, Lt. Murphy said, "My wife and I had tickets to go on vacation in Florida, and I was thinking, 'We're not going to Florida any time soon, and she's going to be pissed.'"

It's funny how our minds work and what things we choose to focus on when we're under duress. With Lt. Murphy it was the thought of his wife being disappointed, and that was something he was not willing to let happen, so he lived. He hung on when others would have given up. Lt. Murphy's survival all came down to his mindset and mental toughness. Somewhere deep down inside, we all have that overpowering will to live. Clawing it out can be difficult sometimes, but I promise you it's there.

When you think of mental toughness your mind may go straight to people who are associated with strength and stamina. Elite military and law enforcement units conjure images of grueling training programs designed to forge the most mentally and physically tough individuals on the planet, but real mental toughness manifests itself in people from all walks of life. When I think of mentally tough people, my mind tends to gravitate toward farmers, specifically my grandfather (Papa). Growing up in the Appalachian Mountains of southern Virginia, I remember Papa getting up hours before the sun was over the horizon and doing more work before breakfast than most people could accomplish in a day. When I asked him why he got up so early, his simple answer was always the same: "Because cows rise early, and they don't milk themselves." That always stuck with me. Sometimes there are things we have to do in life that aren't easy, but we do them anyway. When it comes to farming, if you don't put in the work, you don't eat, and that can get old pretty fast.

Years later, after I had joined the Army, I was in the middle of basic training at Fort Sill, Oklahoma. I had just finished the obstacle course in pretty good time and had always maintained consistently high marksmanship scores. I remember my drill sergeant coming up to me one day and saying, "Damn it, Quesenberry, that's why I love you hillbillies. You can all climb like monkeys, shoot the wings off of a fly, and getting up at five in the morning is like sleeping in to you." I didn't know it at the time, but I think that drill sergeant saw something I didn't even know existed, the early stages of something my Papa had instilled in me years earlier: a positive attitude and mental toughness.

Whether it's a soldier, a farmer, a steel mill worker, or a nurse, mental toughness is a necessity when it comes to being confident and successful. You can look around at those who consistently perform at higher levels and see specific attributes that seem to be more common in the mentally tough.

- They get up early.
- They generally stay in good physical shape.
- They display high levels of motivation.
- They're independent.
- They're consistent.
- They exercise good judgment.
- They're decisive when those around them are hesitant.
- They take responsibility for their actions.
- They can communicate effectively with others.

This is a very short list of attributes associated with mentally tough people. The harder you look, the more you see and the more you appreciate the traits these people exhibit, but what's just as important are the attributes you don't see.

- Mentally tough people don't waste time feeling sorry for themselves.
- They don't give up as soon as they experience a failure.
- They don't avoid tough challenges.
- They don't waste their energy on things they can't control.
- They don't try to please everyone.
- They don't resent the successes of others.
- They don't expect immediate results.

This list isn't all-inclusive, but don't think for a minute that certain groups or individuals have the market cornered on mental toughness. I'm sure you saw several traits you possess, and maybe a few that could use a little work. That brings us to the old "nature versus nurture" argument: is mental toughness something you're born with, or is it something that can be learned and cultivated?

It's true that some people develop high degrees of mental toughness at a very young age; some children grow up in tough situations. Maybe they're from a rough neighborhood, had overly demanding parents, or suffered economic adversities. Living through such situations can play a role in the early development of mental toughness, but it's not a prerequisite.

Over the course of my career, I've found four simple practices that have helped me pull it together from time to time and get my attitude back on track. These four items look deceptively simple on paper but can be incredibly challenging to put into practice.

1. **Get started:** The first step is that simple—pick a task and get started. Whether it's working out in the morning, taking time to read or meditate, spending more quality time with the family, or just knocking out a couple of items on the to-do list, you have to get started. It's not always easy, but once the ball is rolling, it's hard to stop it.
2. **Push yourself:** Never settle for anything other than your absolute best. Once you've given it your all, find a way to make it better. Never stop improving.

3. **Focus on the small victories:** Nothing happens overnight—not weight loss, achieving your fitness goals, or success in business. But you can win small victories every single day that help propel you toward your target. No one decides they're going to run a marathon and the next day they bang out a 26.2-mile run, but you can do a 5K, then work your way up to a 10K, then on to a half-marathon. Eventually, you will make it to your goal, but you have to take the time to appreciate and celebrate the smaller victories along the way.

4. **Don't quit:** This one is probably the most important. Sometimes things get hard, and that sucks, but quitting is never an option. Federal air marshals train extensively for years on how to basically re-hijack an in-flight aircraft against what could be considered impossible odds. Imagine what would happen if things got tough in the middle of all that and the air marshals onboard just quit. It's not an option, so don't even let it cross your mind!

By focusing on these four simple tasks, you can forge a do-or-die mindset that not only carries you through adversity, it can actually help you to thrive in it. Over time these small victories and accomplishments help to build your self-confidence. The more trust you have in your own abilities, the more that confidence begins to manifest itself in your outward appearance. This in turn changes the way you carry yourself and presents more of a hard target to any would-be attacker.

Now let's address a subject nobody wants to talk about: failure. I know, I know—after everything we just covered about mindset and mental toughness you may be thinking, "Why are we even talking about failure? Failure is not an option, right?" Let me put it this way. We never plan to fail. We prepare ourselves mentally and physically for victory in everything we do, and we push ourselves to the absolute limit to see our objectives through to the end. That is the attitude we need to carry with us daily, and it should be the standard operating procedure for achieving every goal we set out to accomplish in life. But the hard truth is, sometimes we fail. Ultimately, how you handle that failure is what will either set you up for future success or put you on the downward spiral of continuous defeat. The route you take is determined by your mindset.

Think for a minute about a failure or defeat you've suffered up to this point. Now, what was the reason for it? Was there not enough time to prepare? Did you not have the proper support? Was there a breakdown in communication or leadership? If you said yes to any of these things, then you are fooling yourself. You're just creating excuses and giving yourself a reason to fail. Failure happens because sometimes we simply go into a situation unprepared. We don't take our time, and we don't look far enough ahead to set up contingency plans so we can correct our course if things go wrong. Our failures have nothing to do with the external issues we try to pin them on and everything to do with our capacity to learn. We all fail at some point, but if you refuse to accept the lessons you are presented with, then you will be doomed to repeat your failures again and again.

I want you to think back to when you learned to ride a bike. You had no real frame of reference for riding, and you probably didn't possess the necessary balance and coordination needed to ride well, but you knew without a doubt that riding a bike was something you were meant to do. Unfortunately, nobody ever gets it right on the first try. I'm sure you suffered your fair share of cuts and scrapes, bruises and embarrassments, but eventually you rode that bike and you got there because you learned from your mistakes and were willing to suffer the pain of failure to do it. Having a positive mindset and being mentally tough is one thing, but being able to maintain that mindset through hardship and adversity is what separates the strong from the weak.

When we look at massively successful people, we tend to focus on the one thing that led to their greatness instead of the numerous failures their accomplishments were built on. The world is filled with people who, despite multiple failures, went on to become top performers in their line of work. Here are a few of my favorite success-from-failure stories. Everyone knows their names, but few people acknowledge the never-quit mindset these individuals possessed to push past their failures and realize their full potential.

- Albert Einstein suffered from a speech impediment until the age of nine. He was expelled from school and was refused admittance into a polytechnic school in Zurich, Switzerland. Despite all this, Albert Einstein went on to develop the theory of general relativity, winning him the Nobel Prize in physics in 1921.
- Walt Disney was in his twenties when he was fired from a Missouri newspaper for "not being creative enough." Then in 1921 Disney founded his first animation studio, Laugh-O-Gram Studio, which went bankrupt within two years. It was only after that failure that Disney decided to move west to pursue his dreams in Hollywood. There, in 1923, he founded the Walt Disney Studio. Over the course of his lifetime, Disney would receive fifty-nine nominations for the Academy Awards and win twenty-two of them.
- Bill Gates was a college dropout whose first business (Traf-O-Data) was a massive failure. He was able to take the lessons he learned from that experience and pioneer his own software company, Microsoft, and by the age of thirty-one became the world's youngest self-made billionaire.
- Michael Jordan was cut from his high school basketball team because his coach didn't think he had the skills necessary to be a successful player. Jordan went on to win six NBA championships and six NBA Finals Most Valuable Player awards, and that's just a small fraction of his total achievements.

Jordan was once asked about the secrets of his success to which he replied, "I've missed more than nine thousand shots in my career. I've lost more than three hundred games. Twenty-six times I've been trusted to take the game winning shot and missed. I've failed over and over and over in my life, and that is why I succeed." That's the attitude we all need to have when it comes to failure. Defeat is never the end of the road. As soon as you accept failure as a sign of completion, then you've pretty much reached your limit in life. You will never be any better than you are at that moment. People who possess a strong winning mindset understand that failure is just part of the game and that no one can be truly great without knowing the sting of defeat. Your level of success in life will be directly proportionate to your ability to learn from your mistakes, so never be afraid to fail. Take it for what it is, learn from it, and move on. That's how I turned my own mindset around after the incident at my children's school and built the defenses necessary to protect my family. Never let past failures cause you to give up on your own security.

There are countless stories of untrained, unprepared people surviving insurmountable odds simply because they refused to give up; they refused to stop trying. When it comes to surviving a violent encounter, your will to win must trump every obstacle you are faced with. Your mindset can literally save your life, and it's the one thing you have absolute control over. Stay positive, stay focused, don't let your fears define your limits, and always maintain a winning mindset.

6.2 Minimizing Distractions

We live in a society obsessed with being somewhere else. By that I mean we choose to occupy our time with thoughts and habits that keep us anywhere but in the moment. Our focus gets split one hundred different ways by electronics, social media, and the constant need to feel "plugged in," so we end up never being able to focus on the task at hand. Nowhere is this more apparent than in the statistics surrounding distracted driving. A study conducted by end.dd.org revealed that texting while driving accounted for 27 percent of all car crashes in 2015. Of those accidents, there were 3,477 deaths and 391,000 injured. Bureau of Justice Statistics, "Drugs and Crime," https://www.enddd.org/the-facts-about-distracted-driving/. Think about that for a minute: that equates to roughly nine deaths per day due to distracted driving, and the numbers have only gone up since 2015.

Distractions are the number-one enemy of situational awareness. Several factors can lead to becoming distracted and taking your focus away from what's important. Things like personal issues at home or work, technological diversions such as smartphones, fatigue, and lack 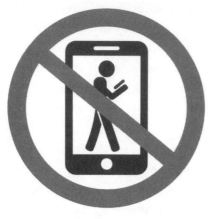 of sleep, excessive noise, or unnecessary conversation. All of these can cause your attention to drift, which in turn can create a lapse in our situational awareness. An old friend of mine once told me that multitasking was impossible. Sure, you can do two things at once, but when you do, you're just doing two things equally bad. That's why it's unsafe to text and drive, or walk down the street while you're posting to Instagram. One task takes away from the effectiveness of the other, and bad things start to happen. When you're out and about, keep your focus where it should be: on your surroundings and your movements. Here are a few precautions you can take to help minimize the likelihood of becoming distracted.

- Get a good night's sleep. Don't leave the house fatigued.
- Iron out any pressing personal issues before you leave home.
- Keep your cell phone in your pocket and only use it when you're in an area you've determined to be safe.
- Don't use headphones or listen to music while you're moving through public areas.
- Don't engage in protracted conversation with strangers.
- Keep your head up and your eyes moving.
- Continually play the what-if game to keep yourself focused on what you're doing.

Make sure that before you set out into the world, you've taken every precaution possible to avoid distraction. It only takes a second for something to go unnoticed, which can create a serious problem down the road.

6.3 Controlling Fear

It's safe to assume Lt. Murphy was experiencing an incredible level of fear and stress during his encounter, but he was able to fight past it. His mental toughness and mindset pushed him through, and he survived. Lt. Murphy is now retired from law enforcement and has received the Congressional Badge of Bravery for his actions during the shooting. More importantly, he finally got to take his wife on that Florida vacation. We all experience fear, and we all have phobias of some sort, but unfortunately fear can easily manifest itself physically. When you experience it, it's clearly visible to others, and in certain situations that can mark you as an easy target. It's crucial we understand what fear is and how it affects us if we ever expect to overcome it and keep it from weakening our defenses.

Phobias are exaggerated, usually inexplicable and illogical fears of objects or situations. Fears manifest themselves in different ways in different people and are often based on past experience, but more often they're completely illogical and without a reasonable explanation. According to research conducted by mentalhealthamerica.net, 10 percent of the population in America suffers from arachnophobia, a fear of spiders. That means that if you threw a spider into a room full of one hundred people, ten of them would lose their minds and run screaming for the nearest exit. There's no real reason for it, they're just deathly afraid of spiders.

Although spiders can be terrifying, there is a situational fear that is far greater. It's what retired Army Lieutenant Colonel David Grossman in his book *On Combat* calls the "Universal Human Phobia," and that's the fear of interpersonal human aggression. This universal phobia affects 95 percent of the population, which means that if you took that same room of one hundred people, and instead of spiders you turned loose a hostile lunatic with a machete, almost all of them would panic. There would be virtually no intelligent thought when it came to resolving the problem. It's a much scarier scenario than a room with a spider in it, and the effects are much more traumatizing. So why are so many more people affected by the fear of human aggression? The answer is because it's personal.

In August of 2005, Hurricane Katrina ripped through New Orleans. There were over 1,800 fatalities, 125 billion dollars in damage, and tens of thousands of people had to abandon their homes. I was there with the Federal Air Marshal Service as part of the rescue effort and saw firsthand the death and devastation the hurricane left behind. Of all the people I helped to evacuate the area, not one of them was mad at the hurricane for the losses they'd suffered. The hurricane was an act of God, and there's no reason a logical human being would take it personally. If, however, someone broke into your home, smashed all your belongings, and beat you and your family so severely you all ended up in the hospital, you would rationally want to hunt that person down and take revenge. Your personal space was invaded, your private things were destroyed, and the ones you love were hurt. The actions taken against you felt personal, and because of that, you have a much different response than if your home had been destroyed in a hurricane.

We humans have an amusing yet ineffective way of insulating ourselves from the fear of personal aggression. From the time we're young, we start to create a story about who we are and what we're capable of. We tell ourselves this story every day, and it begins to define our self-image. You can believe you're a strong, courageous person who would heroically defend the innocent in times of crisis, but when someone angrily confronts you in a parking lot because you cut them off, your stomach will knot up, and your mouth will go dry. You'll stutter out an apology; and when it's all over your hands will shake and you'll be upset with yourself for letting a stranger talk to you that way. Why is that? It's because that sudden aggression from another human being has damaged your precious ego. In mere seconds this person has deconstructed the story you'd been telling yourself; it hurts, and you take it personally. The risk of someone damaging your self-image can generate way more fear than the threat of actual physical harm, but there are ways to counteract this fear, and it all starts with educating yourself about its effects.

What are the steps to recognizing and countering fear? Most importantly, you need to understand fear and how your body reacts to it both physically and mentally. Once you have a basic knowledge of your typical reactions, you can map out ways of minimizing the body's negative responses to it. I want to be perfectly clear here: we will never be able to fully conquer fear or be the master of all things related to confronting violence, but we can train ourselves to a certain level of control. The amount of training you are willing to put yourself through and the level of understanding you strive to achieve dictate your level of control. How far you are willing to push yourself in this process is entirely up to you.

When it comes to physical attacks, the attacker always has the advantage. They get to pick the place, the time, and the method of the attack. They take a rational approach to it, they watch, they rehearse, and they develop contingency plans. They have the element of surprise on their side. The only way to counter this is through early detection and avoidance. Without proper situational awareness, a person is forced to be reactive. The victim finds himself or herself suddenly confronted with danger or violence, and their mind and body go into a tailspin. So many things are happening at once both internally and externally that it becomes hard to comprehend what's happening, much less react to it. That's why it's important to understand the body's natural reactions to stress. Arming yourself with the knowledge of what you'll experience physically and mentally during a violent encounter can give you peace of mind. If you're confronted, you'll know exactly why you feel the way you feel, and you'll know how to counter the adverse effects you're experiencing. More importantly, you'll understand that these natural bodily reactions are there to save your life and that in some cases, you can actually harness their power and use it to your advantage. For instance, once your fear is under some level of control, you can use the adrenaline that's flooded your system to accelerate your escape. We'll now take a closer look at the human nervous system to gain a better understanding of how that works.

The human nervous system has two parts, the sympathetic nervous system (SNS) and the parasympathetic nervous system (PNS). The PNS is commonly referred to as the "rest and digest" system and functions primarily to keep the body's normal operating systems in good working order. But for the purposes of this chapter, the SNS will be our main focus. It is what mobilizes and directs the body's energy resources and prepares you for action. It also triggers your adrenal glands to flood your body with adrenaline. When this happens, certain things occur physically that you'll need to be aware of beforehand. Your heart rate and breathing will speed up so blood and oxygen can be rushed to the muscles, which are being prepped for a fight. Your pupils will dilate, and you could lose your peripheral vision, which causes you to experience "tunnel vision." Tunnel vision is the result of an intense focus on the threat, which leads to an involuntarily decrease in your overall awareness. In high-stress situations, your body may also dull auditory inputs because they're not considered essential to your survival. This is known as auditory exclusion. Many police officers when interviewed after a gunfight reported that they knew they were firing their weapon but can't remember hearing the shots. Their hearing had basically shut down during the fight. There have even been instances where officers thought their weapons were malfunctioning, so instead of returning fire, they were busy trying to fix a nonexistent problem. Another harmful physical side effect is the deterioration of fine motor skills. You experience a tingling in your hands and feet caused by blood vessels constricting, forcing blood away from your extremities and causing it to pool around your internal organs to protect them from damage. This can cause your fingers, arms, and legs to feel week and clumsy. The SNS is also what triggers your fight, flight, or freeze responses. This is an internal survival mechanism as old as time. When confronted with a saber-toothed tiger, the caveman experienced the same adrenaline rush you would experience if confronted by an armed attacker. And both you and the caveman have the same options: you can run, you can fight, or you can stand really still and hope it all just goes away. That last reaction never really works, not with an armed attacker at any rate and certainly not with the tiger. In almost every case, your best options are to run or to fight. The option you pick isn't really up to you, at least not to your rational thinking self. When the SNS is triggered, we tend to go into what I call the "big dumb animal mode." We cease to think rationally, and the big dumb animal inside of us takes over. But like any animal, the big dumb one inside of you can be trained to give the right response. All of these responses triggered by the SNS are natural, and they occur with everyone. The trick is to break the freeze response and act. Once the physical threat is gone, you can begin to relax, your body's systems start to reset, and the intelligent, rational person you were before the confrontation begins to return.

There are four mental states I consider to be toxic and completely counterproductive: fear, confusion, hesitation, and surprise. Each of these mental states is a direct result of stress overload and an inability to properly deal with stress-induced anxiety. I've seen it before—the "martial arts expert" who when confronted by a 250-pound enraged gangbanger finds themselves so completely outmatched that they panic and back down, or the "expert marksman" who at the first sound of gunfire freezes up when the realization sinks in that the bullets are real. No one wants to find themselves outmatched and entirely paralyzed by these toxic mental pitfalls, so that's why we train ourselves in situational awareness, and it's why you picked this book up in the first place. You can improve your odds of surviving a sudden violent attack by taking a couple of simple but effective steps that can prepare your mind and effectively minimize the effects of fear, confusion, hesitation, and surprise. It all starts with becoming comfortable with stress.

When we hear the word inoculation, it tends to conjure up images of childhood vaccinations. Back in the 1700s, an English physician named Edward Jenner discovered that exposing individuals to a less-potent form of a specific disease caused their bodies to create defenses against more severe or even deadly infections further down the road. Inoculation to stress works precisely the same way. By exposing yourself to small levels of stress in training, and gradually increasing those levels, you can effectively train your body to respond more efficiently and to think more clearly under extreme pressure.

Dr. Paul Whitesell was a scientist studying the effects of stress and stress inoculation. His experiments were intended to measure the effectiveness of stress exposure and how it affects performance. Dr. Whitesell started his testing with three groups of rats. All three groups were kept in warm, cozy cages. Dr. Whitesell took the first group of rats from their cages and dropped them into a tub of water to see how long they could swim before drowning. The first group swam for sixty hours. The second group of rats was taken from their comfortable cages, but instead of being dropped directly into the water, Dr. Whitesell held them upside down by their tails to give them a good dose of stress. At some point, the rats would essentially give up; they let the stress get the best of them, and they stopped kicking. That's when they were dropped into the tub of water. That second group of rats only managed to swim for twenty minutes before they drowned. That's a huge difference, right? From sixty hours of swimming to twenty minutes just because they were stressed to their breaking point before they were dropped in the water. The third group of rats was taken from their cages and held upside down until they stopped kicking, but instead of being dropped in the water, they were placed back into their warm, comfortable cages. Dr. Whitesell did this several times a day for several days. On the fourth day, Dr. Whitesell removed the rats from their cages, held them upside down until they stopped kicking, and then dropped them in the water. This third group of rats was able to swim for sixty hours, just like the first group. Unlike the second group, the third group was able to perform normally, despite being exposed to enormous amounts of stress; in short, they had been effectively inoculated. Inoculating humans to stress is very similar. There are plenty of people who are killed every year during violent encounters because they failed to defend themselves adequately; the stress of a sudden violent confrontation was too much for them to handle, and much like the second group of rats, they just gave up. The solution to this problem lies in training. The more you expose yourself to stress the better you're able to control its negative effects, so seek out competent professional self-defense training and expose yourself to a healthy dose of stress from time to time. Now let's take a look at two other techniques you can use to minimize the adverse effects of fear and stress.

The first is combat breathing, Combat breathing is just a more specific method of breathing that when done correctly can significantly reduce your heart rate as well as stress-induced panic and fatigue. Here's how it's done:

1. Inhale through the nose for a count of four. (Actually count it out in your head.)
2. Hold the breath for another count of four.
3. Exhale through the mouth for a count of four.
4. Hold for one last count of four seconds.
5. Repeat.

This technique is also known as box breathing, and it's proven to have a tremendous calming effect even when things are going horribly wrong around you. Combat breathing works because breathing is usually controlled by the sympathetic nervous system; you don't even think about doing it, but when you force yourself to breathe and concentrate on the count, it switches the task to the parasympathetic nervous system, which helps counteract the effects of a stress-induced system overload.

I find myself using this technique in my daily life as a kind of soft reset button. The boss slaps an unrealistic deadline on you . . . combat breathing; the dogs won't stop barking . . . combat breathing; the kids are tearing the house apart . . . combat breathing. It works. Practice it daily when you find yourself stressed or overwhelmed, and you'll instantly see how quickly it can help you to calm down and refocus, and in the event you ever find yourself confronted by violence or injured, it could possibly save your life.

The second technique is known as compartmentalization and is a natural coping mechanism we use to isolate adverse events in our lives and save them for later processing while at the same time focusing on what needs to be done in the moment. Some people view this as a negative trait that allows us to ignore the bad things that happen to us as opposed to dealing with them up front. But compartmentalization can be used as a powerful tool for dealing with fear.

On October 1, 2017, a mass shooter opened fire on thousands of concertgoers on the Las Vegas strip. The gunman fired over one thousand rounds, killing fifty-eight people and injuring more than eight hundred others. When the shooting started, the panic and confusion were instantaneous. People were being killed and wounded in droves without anyone knowing where the shots were coming from because the shooter was attacking from a thirty-second story window 490 yards away from the crowd. With the shooting still going on, several people were able to make it to their cars, but instead of driving away to safety, they managed to make it back into the crowd to help evacuate the injured, driving them to local hospitals. These selfless acts can be directly attributed to the mind's natural ability to compartmentalize. Even in the chaos and confusion of a mass-shooting event, these heroic individuals were able to push aside the negative thoughts of being killed or injured to focus on the evacuation and in the process save countless lives.

Compartmentalization can be used to manage stress and maintain focus in situations ranging from acts of violence to public speaking. What's important to remember is that it's okay to push aside and isolate the immediate emotional reactions you may have to a stress-inducing event for the sake of focusing on the more critical tasks at hand. It's also important to eventually deal with that negativity, but never let it stand in the way of you accomplishing your mission.

6.4 Building Confidence

Self-confidence is an important trait when it comes to managing stress, combating fear, and looking like a hard target. Confidence is also a crucial element in the accomplishment of your goals. Anyone who has a goal in life, whether it's finishing a major project or just getting home safely at night, will need a healthy dose of confidence to achieve that goal. It's what I consider to be the cornerstone of mental toughness and proper mindset.

Confidence is something that you can physically see in people; it manifests itself in the way they walk, speak, and interact with their surroundings. Someone who possesses self-confidence inspires trust in those around them and is often looked to for leadership when situations turn bad. Confidence also tends to dissuade others from taking action against you, especially shady individuals looking for a potential victim. Those with low self-confidence, on the other hand, are typically pushed aside and ignored by others due to their lack of self-assurance; they are also more likely to be the target of violent attacks. People who have low levels of self-confidence often display two particular traits:

1. **They tend to be complainers**: People with low self-confidence often use complaining as a way to shift blame. As opposed to facing their own shortcomings and taking responsibility for their actions, they often whine about the "system" and how if only things were different at some higher level, their performance could improve.

2. **They enjoy being in the spotlight:** People often compensate for their lack of confidence by continually trying to be the center of attention. They do this by speaking louder than those around them. They usually like to show off or brag excessively about their achievements. Don't be fooled by this behavior: the people who genuinely possess self-confidence seldom feel the need to seek approval from others.

Whatever you do, don't confuse confidence with cockiness. Self-confidence isn't easy to come by and is the direct result of life experience. Cockiness, on the other hand, is manufactured and comes from a place of self-doubt. To build a high level of self-confidence takes time, but there are steps you can take to help you get started. Here are a few of the more important ones.

1. **Increase your level of understanding:** The knowledge of how things work, be it physically, mentally, or legally, is invaluable when it comes to building confidence while minimizing fear and indecision. The fear of legal repercussions if you shoot an intruder is just as real as the fear of an actual home invasion. Both concerns are equally dangerous in that they can produce a lack of confidence and cause hesitation. We've already covered the mental and physical chaos caused by sudden violence, and hopefully the knowledge you've gained in those sections helps minimize some of the negative side effects you may experience. Equally as important is a thorough understanding of the law. Take it upon yourself to become an expert in the federal and state laws that govern the use of force in your area. Always stay up to date on local and governmental changes that affect those laws. Confidence in your understanding of the law removes a substantial psychological hurdle when it comes to taking decisive action.

2. **Set goals and see them through:** Another important step in building self-confidence is the setting and achieving of goals. Nothing

helps to build self-confidence more quickly. It doesn't matter if your goals are personal or professional; pick something you want to accomplish and get started on it. Keep your goals realistic and within reach. You may aspire to become a black belt one day but don't know where or how to begin, so a good short-term goal would be to read as much as possible on the subject. Find the martial art that's right for you and best meets your self-defense needs. After you've educated yourself on the basics, start having some conversations with other martial artists and visiting some dojos. Then, sign up for training that interests you and start working on your first belt. No substantial goal is reached overnight, so try not to focus too hard on the finish line. It's the small accomplishments that add up to more significant results, so start realistically and build on your achievements. Before you know it, you can be well on the way to getting that black belt.

Setting goals is easy, but to actually achieve them, you have to do the work. Nothing of importance is ever going to just fall into your lap. If you want something, you have to put in the effort. People who possess true self-confidence push themselves, and they tend to work harder than others when it comes to getting what they need. Once you've achieved something, no matter how small the victory, you've set yourself on the path to positive personal development and with each small success comes increased self-confidence.

3. **Use positive self-talk**: Positive self-talk is another fantastic method of building confidence. We all have an internal monologue and generally "speak" to ourselves anywhere from one thousand to three thousand words per minute. That's a lot, so it stands to reason that the more positive that self-talk is, the better you'll perform. Some beneficial side effects include:
   - Higher self-esteem
   - Reduced levels of stress and anxiety

- Improved self-image
- Physical projection of self-confidence

Those are all pretty significant advantages and help to develop proper levels of confidence and mindset. Positive self-talk also plays an important role in the what-if games. When visualizing specific scenarios, keeping things positive helps you to work your way through to a safe and successful conclusion.

One of the first books I remember reading as a child was *The Little Engine That Could*. In it, a small blue steam engine was tasked with delivering food and toys to a group of children who lived on the other side of a very steep and imposing mountain. No one thought the little engine could do it, but all the way up the mountain the small train kept repeating to itself, "I think I can, I think I can, I think I can." Eventually, the little engine made it over that mountain and delivered its precious cargo to the needy children. I remember this story so vividly because I began using the lessons I learned from reading it almost immediately. When something seemed impossible to me, I thought back to the little blue engine and started telling myself that nothing was impossible. It worked when I was a kid, and it still works now that I'm an adult.

Positive self-talk takes practice. Much like the little engine that could, it has to be repeated over and over before you actually start to believe it. Listen carefully to what you're telling yourself, and when you discover those negative internal thoughts, stop yourself, find a positive way to look at the problem you're facing, and put a constructive spin on the solution. Once you've found your positive voice, internally verbalize that solution to yourself, repeatedly if need be. Over time you'll see that positive self-talk becomes a habit and completely changes the way you tackle the day-to-day problems you're faced with.

All of these things—improving mindset, minimizing distractions, learning to control fear, and building your confidence level—help to reinforce and strengthen your personal defenses. When paired with good situational awareness, they are what allow you to project yourself as a hard target. You'll notice that as you put these elements into practice, you walk a little taller and are more alert to your surroundings. Your movements will convey a sense of intent and purpose, which as you've learned from the Grayson and Stein study, makes you so unappealing to potential predators that they will likely choose to pass you by completely.

Situational Awareness in Action
Julianne Moore Stops a Kidnapper

Julianne Moore was a typical eleven-year-old girl who lived with her parents and younger brother Hayden in the suburbs just outside of Cleveland, Ohio.[1] In the spring of 2019, Julianne and her brother were playing in the front yard near the street while her parents worked in the back. That's when a strange man approached the two children and tried to engage them in conversation. In subsequent interviews with the media, Julianne said, "He started to talk to us, but we really couldn't figure out what he was saying. It was like gibberish, so we really didn't think much of it." Julianne knew to avoid strangers, and something about this man didn't feel right. As the man walked away, Julianne kept a close eye on him. She noticed that he hesitated and circled back toward them. She quickly moved closer to her brother when the stranger lunged for Hayden and tried to pull him away by his arm. At that point, said Julianne, "When he tried to grab my brother, I knew, like this was serious. I just grabbed my brother and went into the backyard because there was no time to panic. You just have to go with it."

The children's father, Joshua Moore, told reporters, "My daughter came running back there with my son, dragging him by the arm and

---

1. *Investigation Discovery*, "Cops: Cleveland Girl, 11, Hero After Saving 6-Year-Old Brother from Attempted Abduction," http://www.investigation discovery.com/crimefeed/survivor-stories/cleveland-girl-saves-little-brother -from-attempted-abduction

said, 'A man tried to abduct Hayden!'" At that point, Joshua ran to the front of the house and confronted the stranger, who continued walking away. He then called the police. Young Julianne had remained calm and observant during the incident and gave the police a detailed description of what the stranger looked like, what he was wearing, and which direction he was headed. Using her report, police located the man nearby, placed him under arrest, and charged him with abduction. Looking back on the incident, Julianne said she was still rattled by what happened but was grateful her parents had taught her to remain calm when faced with an emergency and to always keep an eye on her little brother.

It's crucial that we teach our children to be alert and aware of their surroundings. Julianne's parents went even further by teaching her not to panic during stressful situations and to focus on the things that were most important so she could make clear-headed decisions. Her ability to react to her intuition, remain calm, and remember as much detail about the stranger as possible was instrumental in saving her brother and resolving the situation.

Exercise

Counting Drills

Keeping alert and focused isn't always easy, but there are simple drills to help keep your awareness level up. Below is a list of tasks you can complete mentally any time you're out in public. These simple counting exercises are an effective way to maintain awareness. It takes discipline and conscious effort, but after a while this technique becomes instinctive and greatly improves your chances of spotting a bad situation early.

- When you walk into a room, make it a habit to identify all of the exits.
- Count the number of people in your area, be it a restaurant, train, or parking lot.

- When counting, make sure to look at people's hands. The hands are what can hurt you.
- When walking down the street, periodically stop at a crosswalk or storefront and take a casual look behind you. Count the number of people who appear to be paying attention to what you do.
- When you're in a parking lot, count the number of cars with people sitting in them. How many of those cars are running?

Think back to the target selection exercise you conducted in chapter 1. In step four of the PROD, "Defenses," you asked yourself, "Does this person display any visible signs of defenses? Do they look strong and capable? Are they alert to their surroundings and unlikely to allow an unwanted approach? If so, move on to another person and start over." These simple counting exercises require close observation and concentration. To a potential attacker, this makes you look aware and focused, which makes you a less appealing target.

Key Points
- Improve your mindset
  1. Commit yourself to improving your situational awareness.
  2. Push yourself in your training.
  3. Focus on the small victories.
  4. Don't quit.
- Minimize distractions
  1. Get a good night's sleep. Don't leave the house fatigued.
  2. Iron out any pressing personal issues before you leave home.
  3. Keep your cell phone in your pocket and only use it when you're in an area you've determined to be safe.
  4. Don't use headphones or listen to music while you're moving through public areas.
  5. Don't engage in a protracted conversation with strangers.
  6. Keep your head up and your eyes moving.

7. Continually play the what-if game to keep yourself focused on what you're doing.

- Control fear with combat breathing
  1. Inhale through the nose for a count of four. (Actually count it out in your head.)
  2. Hold the breath for another count of four.
  3. Exhale through the mouth for a count of four.
  4. Hold for one last count of four seconds.
  5. Repeat.
- Build confidence
  1. Increase your level of understanding.
  2. Set goals and see them through.
  3. Use positive self-talk.

7

Putting It All Together

EARLIER, I MENTIONED that after the incident involving my children, I came to the realization that changes needed to be made. Based on my training, I felt I had a pretty good idea of how personal security worked, but I had failed to put all the pieces together. When I took a step back and reevaluated the situation, the root of the problem was staring me right in the face. I had become complacent, and because of that, I had ignored my defenses and left my family vulnerable to attack. That was a hard pill to swallow then, and it's hard to write about even today. I had become what I later referred to as a nine-to-fiver. When I strapped my gun on in the morning and left for the airport, I was 100 percent focused and ready to perform my job. But, at the end of the mission, when I returned home, I developed a habit of dropping my guard and falling into the trap of believing nothing would ever happen to me outside of work. Thirty thousand feet in the air . . . that's where the real bad guys were, right? That was my fatal mistake, and when a real threat presented itself, it came from a direction I had never anticipated. After that day, I began making serious changes, but those changes were incremental; some were made on the spot, but others took time to implement. I still stop once in a while and reevaluate myself from a predator's perspective. I frequently find areas where complacency may have crept in and improvements need to be made. I use the flaws I find to readjust my defenses and strengthen the most vulnerable areas. It's a never-ending process, but if you use the techniques I've outlined in this book, you'll find that improving your situational awareness and hardening your defensive position in life is easier than you think.

We've covered a lot of ground in the last six chapters, and I feel entirely confident that the information I've passed along has opened your eyes to some aspect of situational awareness that, up to this point, you didn't know you were missing. Now you have a pretty good understanding of what factors drive violence and how predators think and act. Given this information, you're now able to look more critically at your own defenses and, through the self-assessment, identify the areas where corrections need to be made. The knowledge of how things work within your environment allows you to accurately establish baselines of behavior and quickly identify events that fall outside the norm. Once something suspicious has been spotted, you can now accurately anticipate the actions of those around you, plan for multiple outcomes, and act decisively when the time comes. That's a pretty impressive set of skills, but when you look at it as a whole, it may seem a little overwhelming. The good news is that all of this information is scalable. You can make a few minor adjustments to your current state of awareness, which will almost instantly increase your level of security, or you can make more significant modifications to your lifestyle, which take more time to master. The choice is up to you. The big question is how do you go about putting what you've learned into practice? Let's review the basics.

1. Heads up! Simply looking around instantly raises your level of awareness and makes you look less appealing to predators.
2. Watch people's hands. If watching people makes you feel a little bit creepy, just make a habit of looking at their hands. The hands are what can hurt you so keep an eye on them.

Those things don't require focused training or years of practice to master. They are simple changes you can implement the next time you leave your house and are enough to greatly improve your chances of spotting danger.

After that, the exercises you've practiced in this book will take your situational awareness to the next level, but these take time and practice. You have to make a concerted effort to incorporate them into your daily routines.

3. Practice performing the seven-second PROD on others to better understand how predators think. What is your perception of those around you? What risk do they pose to you? What observable value do they have? What is their level of defenses?

4. Conduct an honest self-assessment. Determine your current level of security by reviewing the four Ws. Ask yourself who may want to hurt you. What would they want? When and where would they strike?

Understanding the predatory mindset and conducting a self-assessment are crucial in hardening your personal defenses. These two steps take the guesswork out of where your focus should be when you're evaluating your current level of security. This is also an ongoing process. Revisit these steps routinely to make sure you're avoiding complacency and identifying any new threats that may present themselves.

5. Think about where you're going and what the baseline behaviors in that area should be.

6. Remember to remain in a condition-yellow state of awareness. Remain relaxed but alert. This way you can detect problematic situations without burning yourself out through hyper-vigilance.

7. Play environmental KIM's games. Take a quick glance around and make note of what's important.

   a. The number of exits

   b. Possible cover and concealment

   c. Possible improvised weapons

8. Play the what-if game. Frequently assess your situation and ask yourself how you would react in various scenarios. Keep your solutions to these problems simple, but come up with as many realistic options as possible. This is the best way to avoid hesitation should a violent situation present itself.

9. Remember your options. Avoidance first. Then escape and evasion, de-escalation, and finally, confrontation.

Those are the steps you need to take to increase your awareness and improve your personal safety. Use the knowledge you've gained here to take a proactive approach to your own security. Awareness is a state of mind; it's a way of living that has to be cultivated, not only in your own life but in the lives of those you care for. The approach to situational awareness I've given you here works. It's been tested and proven, but for it to be effective, you have to come to the realization that what you have is worth protecting. It's priceless, and you are responsible for it.

Situational Awareness in Action
Uber Hero Keith Avila

Keith Avila is a hard-working husband and father.[1] By day he works as a quinceañera photographer, and at night he makes a little extra money as an Uber driver in Sacramento, California. Keith had only been working with Uber for just under a month, but in that short time he had developed a keen sense of what could be considered normal passenger behavior. As he drove people around, he noticed how they dressed, what they talked about, and how they interacted with each other. He often engaged his passengers in conversation and found that most of his customers were friendly and courteous. One night in December of 2016, Avila picked up three women just outside of Sacramento; their destination was a small hotel in the suburb of Elk Grove only

---

1. Brian Latimer, "Uber Driver Saves Sixteen-Year-Old Girl from Sex Trafficking," NBC News, December 29, 2016, https://www.nbcnews.com/news/amp/ncna701241.

thirteen minutes away. When they got into the car, Avila noticed that something was off about the trio, and as the drive progressed, he began to realize there was nothing routine about this trip.

The first thing Avila noticed was that one of the "women" appeared to be very young. "She appeared to be about twelve years old," Avila later told interviewers. "She had a really short skirt, so you could see all her legs, and it struck me as odd because she was so young and she was dressed like that." After that initial observation, Avila began to pay closer attention. The other two women appeared to be in their early thirties, and they kept very tight control of the younger passenger. When one of the women asked Avila to turn the radio up, he instinctively knew she was trying to mask their conversation. As he listened in, it became apparent that the two older women were coaching the young girl on what she was supposed to do when she arrived at the hotel. Avila said that one of the women told the girl, "First thing you want to do is ask: Do you have any weapons? When you're hugging him just ask, do you have any weapons? Pat him down while you're hugging him. Get the donation first. Before you start touching him, going in there, get the donation first."

All of this information, the inappropriate attire, the odd conversation, and the suspicious destination alerted Avila to the possibility that child sex trafficking may be taking place in his car. He had no idea if the two older women were armed, or if he was in any danger, so when he dropped his passengers off at the hotel, he immediately called the police and told them what had happened. A few minutes later, the police arrived on the scene and arrested the two older women as well as a man who was later identified as the intended "John." The young victim of the sex trafficking ring was recognized as a sixteen-year-old runaway and was later reunited with her family. Avila later told interviewers, "The worst thing I thought would happen when driving Uber is that I would be getting drunk passengers and I would have to handle them. All my life, I thought about people throwing up in the car as the worst-case scenario."

Avila's familiarity with typical passenger conduct had set a baseline for behavior, and he was keenly aware when his passenger's actions rose above that baseline. Not only did his situational awareness save the sixteen-year-old girl from being trafficked, his decision to live stream the police response to the hotel on Facebook had a significant impact on raising awareness of sex trafficking in the community. By the next evening, his video had been viewed over one hundred and twenty thousand times.

Exercise

Six Steps to Spotting Trouble

Now that you're familiar with the basic techniques and exercises used to improve awareness, it's time to put everything together. Any time you're out in public follow these six basic steps and you will dramatically improve your chances of spotting trouble before it has a chance to materialize.

1. Scan the area, look at people's hands, and establish a baseline for behavior.
2. Identify exits and plan the most effective routes for escape.
3. When you enter an area, pay attention to your gut feelings. If something feels wrong or out of place start working out a plan to leave the area if the situation turns bad.
4. Frequently monitor that baseline for changes. If someone's actions rise above the baseline, fall back to step two.
5. Use what-if scenarios to rehearse your reactions to bad situations. Remember to include solutions that address all three elements of personal safety: avoidance, de-escalation, and confrontation.
6. Keep a positive mental attitude. Always see yourself succeeding.

Once you leave the safety of your own home, situational awareness becomes a full-time job. The more you practice these steps the more natural they become. Over time you'll notice that you're taking in more information faster, and without even thinking about it.

Key Points
- Be a hard target.
- Keep your head up.
- Walk with confidence and purpose.
- Maintain awareness.
- Continually visualize "what if" scenarios.
- Know your surroundings.
- Always have an escape plan.

Conclusion

THE CONCEPTS AND TECHNIQUES I've outlined in this book are based on the knowledge and experience I've gained over a twenty-five-year career as a federal law enforcement officer. What I've tried to do here is lay out the principles and techniques I feel are most relevant to personal safety in the hopes that they give you a clear direction when it comes to navigating the complex world of violent encounters. I'd like to close by stressing the importance of regularly practicing what you've learned here. Don't fool yourself into believing that when bad things happen, you will automatically rise to the occasion and save the day. There's a great quote floating around: "You will never rise to the occasion; you will only fall to your level of training." In other words, the ability to keep yourself safe during a violent encounter is not based on some internal superpower that shows up when you need it. Success is based on your mindset and your willingness to practice what you have learned.

As with any training program, you will get out of this book what you put into it. Regardless of how busy your life may be, there will always be time to practice what you've learned here. The more you work through the exercises, the more you'll notice a difference in your level of awareness. Eventually you'll see you're much more in tune with your surroundings. Baseline anomalies and behavioral patterns will become more readily apparent to you, making your ability to preemptively detect danger something that happens on an almost subconscious level. Make sure that when you're practicing these techniques, you're focusing on the proper outcome and using what you see within your environment to plan a safe escape should danger present itself. Getting home safe and sound at the end of each day should always be your ultimate goal. Once you're comfortable with these lessons and they start to become more natural to you, pass your newfound knowledge on to those you care about so they too can enjoy the confidence that comes with knowing they are well prepared. Never forget that you are your own last line of defense. Be mindful, be vigilant, but most of all, be safe!

Appendix

Self-assessment

Who would target you?
List the people who may have grudges against you or raise your suspicion for any reason.

_____

_____

_____

_____

_____

What do they want?
Make a list of the things you have that a predator may find of value. Start with everyday items such as purses, briefcases, backpacks, jewelry, and laptops. Then add to the list things you not only hold valuable but also consider priceless: your family, your home, your pets, and so on.

_____

_____

_____

_____

_____

When would they strike?
Make a list of the times when you feel you would be most vulnerable to attack.

_____

_____

_____

_____

_____

Where would they strike?
Make a list of the places where you feel you may be most vulnerable to an attack.

_____

_____

_____

_____

_____

Strengthen your defenses
Using your self-assessment, continually identify the people, places, and circumstances that could pose a risk to your safety. When you find yourself exposed to one of these risks, make an effort to modify your body language and behavioral patterns to present a hard target to any potential attackers. Use this space to list the possible modifications you could make to help strengthen your personal defenses.

_____

_____

_____

_____

_____

Bibliography

Books

Cooper, Gregory M., and Michael R. King. *Predators: Who They Are and How to Stop Them*. New York: Prometheus Books, 2007.

Dahmer, Lionel. *A Father's Story*. New York: Harper Collins Publishers, 1994.

Dawson, Paul. *Ted Bundy's Girls—Includes My Death Row Interviews with Ted Bundy*. Vistar Pictures Ltd., 2018.

De Becker, Gavin. *The Gift of Fear: Survival Signals That Protect Us from Violence*. New York: Dell Publishing, 1997.

Grossman, Dave, and Loren W. Christensen. *On Combat: The Psychology and Physiology of Deadly Conflict in War and Peace*. Chicago: PPCT Research Publications, 2007.

Miller, Rory. *Facing Violence: Preparing for the Unexpected*. Wolfeboro, NH: YMAA Publication Center, Inc., 2011.

Miller, Rory. *Meditations on Violence: A Comparison of Martial Arts Training and Real World Violence*. Wolfeboro, NH: YMAA Publication Center, Inc., 2008.

Thompson, George J., PhD. *Verbal Judo: The Gentle Art of Persuasion*. New York: Harper Collins Publishers, 1993.

Van Horne, Patrick, and Jason A. Riley. *Left of Bang: How the Marine Corps' Combat Hunter Program Can Save Your Life*. New York: Black Irish Entertainment, LLC, 2011.

Movies

The Bourne Identity. Directed by Doug Liman. 2002. Universal City, CA: NBC Universal.

The Karate Kid. Directed by John G. Avildsen. 1984. Culver City, CA: Columbia Pictures

Web Articles and Videos

Cooper's Colors

Fairburn, Richard. "Coopers Colors: A Simple System for Situational Awareness." PoliceOne.com. Updated July 21, 2017. https://www.policeone.com /police-trainers/articles/2188253-Coopers-colors-A-simple-system-for -situational-awareness/.

Grayson and Stein Study

Grayson, Betty, and Morris I. Stein. "How Assailants Picked Intended Targets." *Journal of Communication* 31 no. 1 (1981): 68–75. https://academic.oup .com/joc/article-abstract/31/1/68/4371921?redirectedFrom=fulltext.

Habits and Motivations of Burglars University of North Carolina at Charlotte. "Through the Eyes of a Burglar: Study Provides Insights on Habits and Motivations, Importance of Security." ScienceDaily. https://www.sciencedaily.com /releases/2013/05/130516160916.htm (accessed November 13, 2019).

Hick's Law

APA Dictionary of Psychology. "Hick's Law." https://dictionary.apa.org/hicks -law.

Lieutenant Brian Murphy Interview

Wyllie, Doug. "Cop Shot 15 Times at Sikh Temple Says, 'Never give up.'" PoliceOne.com. April 22, 2013. https://www.policeone.com/police-heroes/articles /6204982-cop-shot-15-times-at sikh-temple-says-never-give-up/.

OODA Loop

Hightower, Tracy A. "Boyd's OODA Loop and How We Use It." *Tactical Response.* https://www.tacticalresponse.com/blogs/library/18649427-boyd-s-o-o-d-a -loop-and-how-we-use-it.

Phobias

Mental Health America. "Phobias." http://www.mentalhealthamerica.net /conditions/phobias.

Routine Activities Theory

https://www.sciencedirect.com/topics/computer-science/routine-activity -theory.

Stranger and Nonstranger Related Crime

Bureau of Justice Statistics, "Stranger and Nonstranger Crime," https://www
.bjs.gov/index.cfm?ty=tp&tid=941.

Visualization Experiments (Alan Richardson)

Reyes, Alejandro. "Does Visualization Really Work? Here's the Evidence That
It Does." *Expert Enough.* https://expertenough.com/1898/visualization
-works.

Index

9/11, 33, 41

abnormal behavior, 59–60, 79
act (OODA Loop), 46
active shooters, 29, 96
acts of violence, 58
adrenaline, 44, 66, 108–109
adversity, 100–101
aggravated assault, xvii
alarm, 12, 17
al-Qaeda, xv, 3
anticipation, xv, 3
Appalachian Mountains, 97
arachnophobia, 105
armed robbery, 8
assessment, 44, 51, 57, 77, 124. see also
  self-assessment
auditory exclusion, 108–109
Avila, Keith, 124–126
avoidance, 47, 77, 80–85, 107, 124
awareness, basics of, 39–51

baseline anomalies, 55–56, 55–61,
  63–64, 66–69, 70, 72, 93, 130
baseline of behavior, 15–16, 43, 55–59,
  63–64, 70, 72, 79, 93, 122–123, 126
blood, 60, 66, 108–109
body language, 9–10, 15, 17, 34, 82, 88
Bourne Identity, The, xiv
Boyd, John, 45
Brussels, Belgium, xv
Bundy, Ted, 8–9
Bureau of Statistics, xvii
burglaries, 12–13
burglars, 4, 11, 12–13
Burke, Todd, 10

Charlie Hebdo, xv
Cleveland, Ohio, 117
clothing, 10, 81–82
cockiness, 114
combat breathing, 111–112

comfort, level of, 43, 51, 57–58, 78, 82,
  110
communication skills, 88–89
compartmentalization, 112–113
complacency, 3, 29, 121–123
comprehension, 2
Condition Black, 44, 51
Condition Orange, 43–44, 51, 57
Condition Red, 44, 51
Condition White, 43–44, 50–51
Condition Yellow, 43–46, 51, 57–58,
  123
confidence, 7–8, 17, 28, 65.82, 85, 87,
  95, 98, 100, 113–118
confrontation, 6, 14–15, 44, 47–48, 60,
  77, 87, 90–91, 96, 111
confusion, 83, 109
conscious competence, 22
conscious incompetence, 22
contingency plans, 101, 107
Cooper, Gregory M., 10
Cooper, Lieutenant Colonel Jeff, 43
Cooper's Colors, 43–45
correctional officers, 55–56
countering fear, 107
criminals, xvii, 6–15, 19, 43
critical thinking, 39

Dahmer, Jeffrey, 24
Dahmer, Lionel, 24
danger, 7, 21, 39, 42, 58, 62–64, 66–69,
  80, 86, 107
de Becker, Gavin, 69–70
decide (OODA Loop), 46, 49
decision making, 6, 25, 49, 63–64, 77
de-escalation, 47, 77, 87–89, 90, 124,
  126
Defenses (in PROD), 12–13. see also
  personal defenses
denial, 24
Department of Justice, 23
detailed scan, 57–62

deterrents, 7, 11–13, 27, 93
DiPietro, Danny, 69–70
discipline, 31, 118
Disney, Walt, 102
distracted driving, 103
distractions, 12, 28, 64, 93, 103–105
dominant, 78
Douglas County, Colorado, 42

early detection, 95, 107
ego, 5–6, 107
Einstein, Albert, 102
element of surprise, 107
Elizabeth, New Jersey, 91
emotion, 6
end.dd.org, 103
environmental cues, 39
escape, 43, 47–48, 50, 59, 62, 83, 85–86, 90
escape routes, 50, 59, 83, 85–86
Europe, 82
evasion, 85–86
excessive sweating, 61
eye contact, 10, 27–28, 59, 83, 89

Facing Violence: Preparing for the Unexpected, 4
failure, 100–103
failure to monitor the baseline, 63–64
fear, 60–61, 65–66, 103, 105–113, 114
Federal Air Marshal Service, 3, 21, 41, 47, 62, 78, 106
federal air marshals, xiii, xv, 19, 29, 58, 100
federal prison, 5, 55
fight, flight, or freeze responses, 44, 51, 60, 109
fight, willingness to put up a, 10, 12, 17
fine motor skills, 108
focus lock, 64
four stages of learning, 21–22
Four Ws (who, what, when, and where), 19, 28, 123

Gates, Bill, 102
Gift of Fear, The, 67
goosebumps, 66
gray man, 81
Grayson, Betty, 8
Grayson and Stein study, 8–9, 14–15, 80, 117
Grossman, Lieutenant Colonel David, 105
grudges, 22, 24
Grundl, Joey, 48–49
gunfights, 108

hands, 58, 65, 93, 119, 122
hard targets, 7, 10, 14, 34, 39, 80, 100, 113, 117
heavier-than-usual breathing, 60
hesitation, 28, 109–110, 114, 124
Hick, William Edmond, 46
Hick's Law, 46–48
hijackings, 3–4, 41
homicide, 41
House of Parliament, xvi
Howell, Michigan, 69
human nervous system, 108–109
Hurricane Katrina, 106
hyper-vigilance, 4, 40, 43, 123

identifying, awareness and, 57–62
impeding your movement, 59
inappropriate clothing, 59
inexplicable presence, 58, 68
initial scan, 54–57, 62, 78
inmates, 5, 8–9, 56
INS, 15
intelligence operatives, 81
intent, 60, 79, 90
intuition, 66–69
Islamic State, xv

Jenner, Edward, 110
Jordan, Michael, 102

Karate Kid, The, 90

KIM's Game, 53–54, 61–62, 70–72
King, Michael R., 10

Las Vegas Strip, 41, 112
law enforcement, 53, 59–60, 79
LAX airport, 15
leadership, 113
LEAPS (Listen, Empathize, Ask, Paraphrase, Summarize), 89
Left of Bang, 78
levels of awareness, 42–45
Little Engine That Could, The, 116
London Bridge, xvi

manslaughter, xvii
McHoes, Thomas, 10
means, 79
mental rehearsals, 30, 31
mental toughness, 97–100, 105, 113
mentalhealthamerica.net, 105
Miller, Rory, 4
mindset, improving, 96–103, 105, 113, 116, 117
minimizing distractions, 12, 28, 95, 103–105, 117
Minskoff Theatre, 32
money, 4–5, 84–85
Moore, Joshua, 117–118
Moore, Julianne, 117–118
Morris-Stein study, 8–9
multitasking, 104
murder, xvii, 23, 82
Murphy, Lieutenant Brian, 96–97, 105
muscle memory, 31

national crime survey, 99
nature versus nurture, 99
Nesmeth, James, 30
New Orleans, 106
New York City, 8, 32, 41, 92
normalcy bias, 64

observable value (in PROD), 12, 14, 17, 25, 28, 82
observe (in OODA Loop), 45

Omaha, Nebraska, 29
On Combat, 105
OODA Loop, 45, 46, 49
opportunity, 80
orient (in OODA Loop), 45, 46, 49
outward signs of security, 7, 12, 17
oxygen, 60, 108

Papa, 97
parasympathetic nervous system (PNS), 108, 112
Paris, France, xv, 61
Parker, Lee, 91–92
passports, 15
patterns, xvii, 17, 18, 26, 34, 42, 54–56, 92, 93, 130
pedestrian behaviors, 14
perception (in PROD), 8–10, 11, 17, 28, 40–42
perception versus reality, 40–42
personal defenses, 18–20, 22, 33–34, 40
phobias, 105–106
physiological reactions, 60–61
planning, 39, 44, 45, 49, 86
Port Angeles, 15–16
position of advantage, seeking, 59
positioning, 80, 83
posture, 8, 10, 17, 88, 92, 93
posturing, 60
predatorial mindset, 14, 19, 27
predator's perspective, 13–15
Predators: Who They Are and How to Stop Them, 10
predatory behaviors, 3–15
pre-incident indicators, 42, 58–62, 68–69, 79, 117, 123
process predators, 4, 25, 87
protectors, 29–32

random acts of violence, 29
rape, xvii, 8, 10
reactionary gap, 46–48
reactionary times, 40, 46, 49–50, 92, 93

resource predators, 4, 25, 87
Ressam, Ahmed, 15–16
Richardson, Alan, 31
Riley, Jason A., 78
risk (in PROD), 10–14, 17
risk versus reward, 7, 16
robbery, xvii, 8, 23
roleplaying, 27–29, 88
route planning, 92–93
routine activities theory, 26–27
Rule of Three, 60, 78

Sacramento, California, 124
San Bruno, California, 41
security, outward signs of, 7, 12, 13
self-assessment, 19–32, 33–34, 123, 131–132
self-confidence, 100, 113–117
self-defense, 47–48, 80, 115
self-defense training, 47–48, 115
self-image, 5, 106–107, 116
self-talk, positive, 115–116
seven-second PROD, 7–13, 17, 19, 27, 29, 123
sexual predators, xii, 8, 10
Shahzad, Faisal, 33
Sheboygan County, Wisconsin, 48
Sikh temple shooting, 96
social media, 14, 25, 103
soft targets, 7, 14, 16, 65, 80–81, 85, 95, 104
strangers, 23–25
street crime, 12
stress
stress exposure, 110
stress inoculation, 110
universal physiological reactions to, 60–61, 79, 107
stride, 9–10
submissiveness, 78
sudden change of movement, 59
suicide bombers, xv, 83
surprise, 90, 107, 109, 110

surroundings, 43, 51, 53, 57–58, 63, 64, 80, 81, 85, 86, 117, 118, 119
surveillance, xiii
sympathetic nervous system (SNS), 108, 112

target glancing, 59
target selection, 7, 10, 16, 17–18, 119
tension, appearance of, 60
territory, 119
terrorists, xv, 3, 21, 33, 41, 42, 61, 83
Thompson, George, 88
tunnel vision, 108

uncomfortable (mode of behavior), 78
unconscious competence, 22
unconscious incompetence, 21
Uniform Crime Report (UCR), FBI's, xvi–xvii
unsolicited attempts at conversation, 59, 68

value, 12–14, 17, 25, 26, 28, 82, 84, 85
Van Horn, Patrick, 78
Verbal Judo Institute, 88
Verbal Judo: The Gentle Art of Persuasion, 88
Victoria, Canada, 15
violence, 4, 6, 48, 66, 80, 81, 107
violent crime, motiving factors of, 4–6
visible defenses, 7, 13, 17, 26, 79, 119
visualization, 30–32, 116
visualization techniques, 31
vulnerabilities, 8–9, 19, 25–27

Westminster Bridge, xvi
Westroads Mall, 29
what-if games, 30–31, 49–50, 64, 78, 88, 116, 124, 126
White, Ivan, 92
Whitesell, Paul, 110

Zurich, Switzerland, 102

About the Author

GARY QUESENBERRY was born in the Blue Ridge Mountains of Virginia. His love of the outdoors and patriotic spirit led him to enlist in the United States Army where he served as an artilleryman during Operation Desert Storm. Gary later became a career federal air marshal and trainer where he has devoted his life to studying violence and predatory behavior. Now Gary serves as the CEO of Q-Series LLC and has developed numerous basic- and advanced-level training courses focused on mental toughness, marksmanship, and defensive tactics. As a competitive pistol shooter, Gary has been featured on the History Channel's hit television series *Top Shot, Season 3* and *Top Shot All-Stars*. He has an extensive background in domestic and foreign counterterror training and has worked in both the private and corporate sectors to help educate others on the importance of situational awareness and personal safety through his "Heads Up" training program.

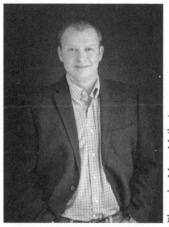

Photo by Mary Mcilvaine

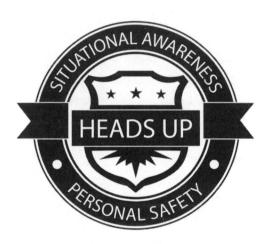

www.garyquesenberry.com

BOOKS FROM YMAA

101 REFLECTIONS ON TAI CHI CHUAN
108 INSIGHTS INTO TAI CHI CHUAN
A SUDDEN DAWN: THE EPIC JOURNEY OF BODHIDHARMA
A WOMAN'S QIGONG GUIDE
ADVANCING IN TAE KWON DO
ANALYSIS OF SHAOLIN CHIN NA 2ND ED
ANCIENT CHINESE WEAPONS
THE ART AND SCIENCE OF STAFF FIGHTING
THE ART AND SCIENCE OF STICK FIGHTING
ART OF HOJO UNDO
ARTHRITIS RELIEF, 3D ED.
BACK PAIN RELIEF, 2ND ED.
BAGUAZHANG, 2ND ED.
BRAIN FITNESS
CARDIO KICKBOXING ELITE
CHIN NA IN GROUND FIGHTING
CHINESE FAST WRESTLING
CHINESE FITNESS
CHINESE TUI NA MASSAGE
CHOJUN
COMPLETE MARTIAL ARTIST
COMPREHENSIVE APPLICATIONS OF SHAOLIN CHIN NA
CONFLICT COMMUNICATION
CUTTING SEASON: A XENON PEARL MARTIAL ARTS THRILLER
DAO DE JING
DAO IN ACTION
DEFENSIVE TACTICS
DESHI: A CONNOR BURKE MARTIAL ARTS THRILLER
DIRTY GROUND
DR. WU'S HEAD MASSAGE
DUKKHA HUNGRY GHOSTS
DUKKHA REVERB
DUKKHA, THE SUFFERING: AN EYE FOR AN EYE
DUKKHA UNLOADED
ENZAN: THE FAR MOUNTAIN, A CONNOR BURKE MARTIAL ARTS
    THRILLER
ESSENCE OF SHAOLIN WHITE CRANE
EVEN IF IT KILLS ME
EXPLORING TAI CHI
FACING VIOLENCE
FIGHT BACK
FIGHT LIKE A PHYSICIST
THE FIGHTER'S BODY
FIGHTER'S FACT BOOK
FIGHTER'S FACT BOOK 2
THE FIGHTING ARTS
FIGHTING THE PAIN RESISTANT ATTACKER
FIRST DEFENSE
FORCE DECISIONS: A CITIZENS GUIDE
FOX BORROWS THE TIGER'S AWE
INSIDE TAI CHI
THE JUDO ADVANTAGE
THE JUJI GATAME ENCYCLOPEDIA
KAGE: THE SHADOW, A CONNOR BURKE MARTIAL ARTS
    THRILLER
KARATE SCIENCE
KATA AND THE TRANSMISSION OF KNOWLEDGE
KRAV MAGA COMBATIVES
KRAV MAGA PROFESSIONAL TACTICS
KRAV MAGA WEAPON DEFENSES
LITTLE BLACK BOOK OF VIOLENCE
LIUHEBAFA FIVE CHARACTER SECRETS
MARTIAL ARTS ATHLETE
MARTIAL ARTS INSTRUCTION
MARTIAL WAY AND ITS VIRTUES
MASK OF THE KING
MEDITATIONS ON VIOLENCE
MERIDIAN QIGONG EXERCISES
MIND/BODY FITNESS
MINDFUL EXERCISE
THE MIND INSIDE TAI CHI
THE MIND INSIDE YANG STYLE TAI CHI CHUAN
NATURAL HEALING WITH QIGONG
NORTHERN SHAOLIN SWORD, 2ND ED.
OKINAWA'S COMPLETE KARATE SYSTEM: ISSHIN RYU

THE PAIN-FREE BACK
PAIN-FREE JOINTS
POWER BODY
PRINCIPLES OF TRADITIONAL CHINESE MEDICINE
THE PROTECTOR ETHIC
QIGONG FOR HEALTH & MARTIAL ARTS 2ND ED.
QIGONG FOR LIVING
QIGONG FOR TREATING COMMON AILMENTS
QIGONG MASSAGE
QIGONG MEDITATION: EMBRYONIC BREATHING
QIGONG MEDITATION: SMALL CIRCULATION
QIGONG, THE SECRET OF YOUTH: DA MO'S CLASSICS
QUIET TEACHER: A XENON PEARL MARTIAL ARTS THRILLER
RAVEN'S WARRIOR
REDEMPTION
ROOT OF CHINESE QIGONG, 2ND ED.
SAMBO ENCYCLOPEDIA
SCALING FORCE
SELF-DEFENSE FOR WOMEN
SENSEI: A CONNOR BURKE MARTIAL ARTS THRILLER
SHIHAN TE: THE BUNKAI OF KATA
SHIN GI TAI: KARATE TRAINING FOR BODY, MIND, AND SPIRIT
SIMPLE CHINESE MEDICINE
SIMPLE QIGONG EXERCISES FOR HEALTH, 3RD ED.
SIMPLIFIED TAI CHI CHUAN, 2ND ED.
SOLO TRAINING
SOLO TRAINING 2
SPOTTING DANGER BEFORE IT SPOTS YOU
SUMO FOR MIXED MARTIAL ARTS
SUNRISE TAI CHI
SURVIVING ARMED ASSAULTS
TAE KWON DO: THE KOREAN MARTIAL ART
TAEKWONDO BLACK BELT POOMSAE
TAEKWONDO: A PATH TO EXCELLENCE
TAEKWONDO: ANCIENT WISDOM FOR THE MODERN WARRIOR
TAEKWONDO: DEFENSE AGAINST WEAPONS
TAEKWONDO: SPIRIT AND PRACTICE
TAI CHI BALL QIGONG: FOR HEALTH AND MARTIAL ARTS
TAI CHI BALL WORKOUT FOR BEGINNERS
THE TAI CHI BOOK
TAI CHI CHIN NA: THE SEIZING ART OF TAI CHI CHUAN,
    2ND ED.
TAI CHI CHUAN CLASSICAL YANG STYLE, 2ND ED.
TAI CHI CHUAN MARTIAL POWER, 3RD ED.
TAI CHI CONNECTIONS
TAI CHI DYNAMICS
TAI CHI FOR DEPRESSION
TAI CHI IN 10 WEEKS
TAI CHI QIGONG, 3RD ED.
TAI CHI SECRETS OF THE ANCIENT MASTERS
TAI CHI SECRETS OF THE WU & LI STYLES
TAI CHI SECRETS OF THE WU STYLE
TAI CHI SECRETS OF THE YANG STYLE
TAI CHI SWORD: CLASSICAL YANG STYLE, 2ND ED.
TAI CHI SWORD FOR BEGINNERS
TAI CHI WALKING
TAIJIQUAN THEORY OF DR. YANG, JWING-MING
TAO OF BIOENERGETICS
TENGU: THE MOUNTAIN GOBLIN, A CONNOR BURKE MARTIAL
    ARTS THRILLER
TIMING IN THE FIGHTING ARTS
TRADITIONAL CHINESE HEALTH SECRETS
TRADITIONAL TAEKWONDO
TRAINING FOR SUDDEN VIOLENCE
TRUE WELLNESS
TRUE WELLNESS: THE MIND
TRUE WELLNESS FOR YOUR HEART
THE WARRIOR'S MANIFESTO
WAY OF KATA
WAY OF SANCHIN KATA
WAY TO BLACK BELT
WESTERN HERBS FOR MARTIAL ARTISTS
WILD GOOSE QIGONG
WINNING FIGHTS
WISDOM'S WAY

DVDS FROM YMAA

ADVANCED PRACTICAL CHIN NA IN-DEPTH
ANALYSIS OF SHAOLIN CHIN NA
ATTACK THE ATTACK
BAGUA FOR BEGINNERS 1
BAGUA FOR BEGINNERS 2
BAGUAZHANG: EMEI BAGUAZHANG
BEGINNER QIGONG FOR WOMEN 1
BEGINNER QIGONG FOR WOMEN 2
BEGINNER TAI CHI FOR HEALTH
CHEN STYLE TAIJIQUAN
CHEN TAI CHI FOR BEGINNERS
CHIN NA IN-DEPTH COURSES 1—4
CHIN NA IN-DEPTH COURSES 5—8
CHIN NA IN-DEPTH COURSES 9—12
FACING VIOLENCE: 7 THINGS A MARTIAL ARTIST MUST KNOW
FIVE ANIMAL SPORTS
FIVE ELEMENTS ENERGY BALANCE
INFIGHTING
INTRODUCTION TO QI GONG FOR BEGINNERS
JOINT LOCKS
KNIFE DEFENSE: TRADITIONAL TECHNIQUES AGAINST A
    DAGGER
KUNG FU BODY CONDITIONING 1
KUNG FU BODY CONDITIONING 2
KUNG FU FOR KIDS
KUNG FU FOR TEENS
LOGIC OF VIOLENCE
MERIDIAN QIGONG
NEIGONG FOR MARTIAL ARTS
NORTHERN SHAOLIN SWORD : SAN CAI JIAN, KUN WU JIAN,
    QI MEN JIAN
QI GONG 30-DAY CHALLENGE
QI GONG FOR ANXIETY
QI GONG FOR ARMS, WRISTS, AND HANDS
QIGONG FOR BEGINNERS: FRAGRANCE
QI GONG FOR BETTER BREATHING
QI GONG FOR CANCER
QI GONG FOR ENERGY AND VITALITY
QI GONG FOR HEADACHES
QI GONG FOR HEALING
QI GONG FOR HEALTHY JOINTS
QI GONG FOR HIGH BLOOD PRESSURE
QIGONG FOR LONGEVITY
QI GONG FOR STRONG BONES
QI GONG FOR THE UPPER BACK AND NECK
QIGONG FOR WOMEN
QIGONG FOR WOMEN WITH DAISY LEE
QIGONG MASSAGE
QIGONG MINDFULNESS IN MOTION
QIGONG: 15 MINUTES TO HEALTH
SABER FUNDAMENTAL TRAINING
SAI TRAINING AND SEQUENCES
SANCHIN KATA: TRADITIONAL TRAINING FOR KARATE POWER
SCALING FORCE
SHAOLIN KUNG FU FUNDAMENTAL TRAINING: COURSES 1 & 2
SHAOLIN LONG FIST KUNG FU: ADVANCED SEQUENCES 1
SHAOLIN LONG FIST KUNG FU: ADVANCED SEQUENCES 2
SHAOLIN LONG FIST KUNG FU: BASIC SEQUENCES
SHAOLIN LONG FIST KUNG FU: INTERMEDIATE SEQUENCES
SHAOLIN SABER: BASIC SEQUENCES
SHAOLIN STAFF: BASIC SEQUENCES
SHAOLIN WHITE CRANE GONG FU BASIC TRAINING: COURSES
    1 & 2

SHAOLIN WHITE CRANE GONG FU BASIC TRAINING: COURSES
    3 & 4
SHUAI JIAO: KUNG FU WRESTLING
SIMPLE QIGONG EXERCISES FOR HEALTH
SIMPLE QIGONG EXERCISES FOR ARTHRITIS RELIEF
SIMPLE QIGONG EXERCISES FOR BACK PAIN RELIEF
SIMPLIFIED TAI CHI CHUAN: 24 & 48 POSTURES
SIMPLIFIED TAI CHI FOR BEGINNERS 48
SUNRISE TAI CHI
SUNSET TAI CHI
SWORD: FUNDAMENTAL TRAINING
TAEKWONDO KORYO POOMSAE
TAI CHI BALL QIGONG: COURSES 1 & 2
TAI CHI BALL QIGONG: COURSES 3 & 4
TAI CHI BALL WORKOUT FOR BEGINNERS
TAI CHI CHUAN CLASSICAL YANG STYLE
TAI CHI CONNECTIONS
TAI CHI ENERGY PATTERNS
TAI CHI FIGHTING SET
TAI CHI FIT: 24 FORM
TAI CHI FIT: FLOW
TAI CHI FIT: FUSION BAMBOO
TAI CHI FIT: FUSION FIRE
TAI CHI FIT: FUSION IRON
TAI CHI FIT: HEART HEALTH WORKOUT
TAI CHI FIT IN PARADISE
TAI CHI FIT: OVER 50
TAI CHI FIT OVER 50: BALANCE EXERCISES
TAI CHI FIT OVER 50: SEATED WORKOUT
TAI CHI FIT OVER 60: GENTLE EXERCISES
TAI CHI FIT OVER 60: HEALTHY JOINTS
TAI CHI FIT OVER 60: LIVE LONGER
TAI CHI FIT: STRENGTH
TAI CHI FIT: TO GO
TAI CHI FOR WOMEN
TAI CHI FUSION: FIRE
TAI CHI QIGONG
TAI CHI PUSHING HANDS: COURSES 1 & 2
TAI CHI PUSHING HANDS: COURSES 3 & 4
TAI CHI SWORD: CLASSICAL YANG STYLE
TAI CHI SWORD FOR BEGINNERS
TAI CHI SYMBOL: YIN YANG STICKING HANDS
TAIJI & SHAOLIN STAFF: FUNDAMENTAL TRAINING
TAIJI CHIN NA IN-DEPTH
TAIJI 37 POSTURES MARTIAL APPLICATIONS
TAIJI SABER CLASSICAL YANG STYLE
TAIJI WRESTLING
TRAINING FOR SUDDEN VIOLENCE
UNDERSTANDING QIGONG 1: WHAT IS QI? • HUMAN QI
    CIRCULATORY SYSTEM
UNDERSTANDING QIGONG 2: KEY POINTS • QIGONG
    BREATHING
UNDERSTANDING QIGONG 3: EMBRYONIC BREATHING
UNDERSTANDING QIGONG 4: FOUR SEASONS QIGONG
UNDERSTANDING QIGONG 5: SMALL CIRCULATION
UNDERSTANDING QIGONG 6: MARTIAL QIGONG BREATHING
WATER STYLE FOR BEGINNERS
WHITE CRANE HARD & SOFT QIGONG
YANG TAI CHI FOR BEGINNERSS
WUDANG KUNG FU: FUNDAMENTAL TRAINING
WUDANG SWORD
WUDANG TAIJIQUAN
XINGYIQUAN

more products available from . . .
YMAA Publication Center, Inc. 楊氏東方文化出版中心
1-800-669-8892 • info@ymaa.com • www.ymaa.com

YMAA
PUBLICATION CENTER